Guidelines for AUDIOLOGIC SCREENING

American Speech-Language-Hearing Association
Panel on Audiologic Assessment

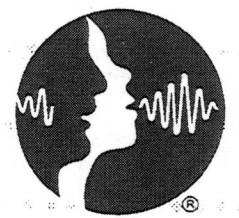

AMERICAN
SPEECH-LANGUAGE-
HEARING
ASSOCIATION

General Information

Guidelines for Audiologic Screening is published by the American Speech-Language-Hearing Association to support practitioners' efforts to provide quality and effective service delivery.

Published by the American Speech-Language-Hearing Association
10801 Rockville Pike, Rockville, MD 20852-3279

Copyright 1997 by the American Speech-Language-Hearing Association

ISBN: 0-910329-96-6

Copies may be ordered from:
ASHA Fulfillment Operations
10801 Rockville Pike
Rockville, MD 20852-3279
(301) 897-5700, ext. 218

Table of Contents

Acknowledgments

The development of guidelines as policy of the American Speech-Language-Hearing Association (ASHA) is a dynamic and democratic process: Member volunteers expert in the topic are enlisted to author a draft document, consider the peer review solicited from colleagues, and incorporate consensus opinion and preferred practice into a final submission for Executive Board and Legislative Council action. The Panel on Audiologic Assessment did just this: Members pondered significant data, resolved a number of controversial matters, and compiled Guidelines on Audiologic Screening that offer a framework for provision of screening for hearing impairment, disability, and disorder across the life span, from newborns to seniors. A heartfelt thanks to Panel members (Chie Craig, chair; pediatric working group: coordinator Deborah Hayes, with Kathryn Beauchaine, Stefanie Bronson, Robert Nozza, Anne Marie Tharpe, and Judith Widen; adult working group: coordinator Sabina Schwan, with Gary Jacobson and Wayne Olsen; and Larry Higdon, Vice President for Professional Practices in Audiology) for completing an extremely difficult task with enthusiasm, care, and a comprehensive knowledge of pertinent research.

Steadfast editors facilitated the shaping of this document through a large number of iterations: in the early stages Penny Watts and Ellen Caswell provided style and "fine tuning"; Jude Langsam managed the final editing and desktop and product preparation with skill and appreciated haste. Tarja Carter contributed her unique flair for graphic design.

Audiologic screening guidelines are frequently requested by ASHA members as well as program administrators and professionals responsible for establishment and implementation of such programs for children and/or adults. ASHA is pleased to provide this policy document to enhance primary and secondary prevention programs for the identification and treatment of persons at risk for or with hearing impairment, disability, and/or disorder.

Evelyn Cherow
ASHA, Audiology Division
Ex officio, ASHA Panel on Audiologic Assessment

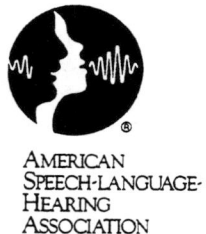

AMERICAN
SPEECH-LANGUAGE-
HEARING
ASSOCIATION

Guidelines for Audiologic Screening

I. Background

The Guidelines for Audiologic Screening were developed by the American Speech-Language-Hearing Association (ASHA) Panel on Audiologic Assessment and adopted as ASHA policy by the Legislative Council in November 1996 (LC19-96). Members of the Panel on Audiologic Assessment are Chie Craig, chair; pediatric working group: coordinator Deborah Hayes, with Kathryn Beauchaine, Stefanie Bronson, Robert Nozza, Anne Marie Tharpe, and Judith Widen; adult working group: coordinator Sabina Schwan, with Gary Jacobson and Wayne Olsen; Evelyn Cherow, ex officio; and Larry Higdon, Vice President for Professional Practices in Audiology, serving as the monitoring Executive Board officer.

These guidelines supersede the following ASHA policies and report:

* *American Speech-Language-Hearing Association. (1985, May). Guidelines for identification audiometry. Asha, 27, 49–53.*

* *American Speech-Language-Hearing Association. (1989, March). Audiologic screening of newborn infants who are at risk for hearing impairment. Asha, 31, 89–92.*

* *American Speech-Language-Hearing Association. (1990, April). Guidelines for screening for hearing impairment and middle-ear disorders. Asha, 32 (Suppl. 2), 17–24.*

* *American Speech-Language-Hearing Association. (1992, August). Report: Considerations in screening adults/older persons for handicapping hearing impairment. Asha, 34, 81–87.*

ASHA's strong commitment to the prevention and early detection of audiologic disorders is evidenced by Article II of the ASHA Bylaws that states: (one of) "the purposes of this organization shall be to ... promote investigation and prevention of disorders of human communication." Primary prevention includes altering susceptibility or reducing exposure to causes of hearing loss. Audiologic screening serves a secondary prevention function; that is, if a hearing disorder, impairment, or disability is detected and treated early, potential hearing-related problems can be prevented or ameliorated. Screening refers to a specific way to indicate need for further assessment for a disorder, impairment, or disability.

Several ASHA policy documents pertinent to audiologic screening in children and adults exist (ASHA, 1995). These guidelines and position statements are products of the efforts of several ASHA committees. Focused on screening for specific conditions or in specific populations, some of the extant guidelines continue to provide valuable information. A review of the documents, however, revealed that some guidelines overlapped, others needed updating and revision, and as a whole, the guidelines did not address audiologic screening across the life span (ASHA, 1985, 1989, 1990, 1991b; Joint Committee on Infant Hearing, 1994).

In 1993, the Ad Hoc Committee on Screening for Hearing Impairment, Handicap, and Middle Ear Disorders recommended the establishment of a mechanism within ASHA to "monitor screening guidelines and protocols for hearing impairment, disability, and middle ear disorders" (ASHA, 1995). As a result, ASHA established the Panel on Audiologic Assessment in 1995 with the following charge:

> Review and update of pertinent ASHA policies and reports and the development of ASHA audiologic assessment and screening guidelines with consideration of traditional screening and diagnostic audiometry, auditory evoked potentials, otoacoustic emissions, and acoustic immittance procedures for pediatric and adult populations.

Based on previous committees' recommendations, current research findings, and changes in screening technology, the Panel determined that new, updated, and consolidated audiologic screening guidelines should be developed for all age groups and contained in a single document.

Early in its deliberations, the Panel agreed that, to maintain consistency across guidelines, important comprehensive design, development, and professional issues needed to be addressed. The Panel's preliminary discussions, therefore, focused on the following issues: (a) principles of screening; (b) test performance; (c) program development, management, and follow-up; (d) definitions of disorder, impairment, and disability; and (e) organizational framework. The following section contains the Panel's resolutions regarding each of these issues.

A. Principles of Screening

These ASHA screening guidelines represent the official policy of the Association and adhere to generally accepted principles for the detection of a disease (ASHA, 1995):

Purpose of Screening

The purpose of screening is to detect, among apparently healthy persons, those individuals who demonstrate a greater probability for having a disease or condition, so they may be referred for further evaluation.

Importance of the Disease

The greater the potential burden a disease represents to the individual and society, the greater the impetus to screen.

Diagnostic Criteria

For a screening program to be successful, there must be a clear and measurable definition of the disease one is attempting to identify through screening.

Treatment

Before a screening program is implemented, it is necessary to demonstrate that treatments are available, effective, and shown to alter the natural history of the disease.

Reaching Those Who Could Benefit

Screening programs are particularly valuable to those individuals who might benefit from early detection and intervention. Public policy can influence how well screening programs succeed in reaching the appropriate population.

Availability of Resources/Compliance

Effective and available diagnostic and treatment referral resources for the disease must be established prior to screening, as the value of screening depends on competent follow-up.

Appropriateness of the Test

Ideally a screening test should be easy to administer, comfortable for the patient, short in duration, and inexpensive. The test must also meet certain performance criteria; that is, it must be sensitive and specific.

Screening Program Evaluation

Screening programs can and should be evaluated. Any recommended protocol should be based on data that demonstrate that those who are identified through screening have better outcomes than those not screened. Program costs can be estimated.

Because persons involved in audiologic screening should be familiar with these screening principles, important relevant references with more detailed discussions are provided (ASHA, 1992, 1994; Cadman, Chambers, Feldman, & Sackett, 1984; Feightner, 1992; Frankenburg, 1974; Hyde, Davidson, & Alberti, 1991; Swets, 1988; Thorner & Remein, 1982; Turner, 1991, 1992a, 1992b; Turner & Cone-Wesson, 1992; Weinstein & Fineberg, 1980).

B. Screening Test Performance

The appropriate selection of a screening test depends, in part, on the test's performance in separating those with the target condition from those without the target condition. Whatever screening test is selected, a single cutoff value (the test criterion) must be chosen. The outcome of the screening is one of two possibilities: pass or refer.

The Panel selected test criteria based on a number of factors. Tests usually produce scores over a range along a continuum (e.g., hearing thresholds vary along the dB HL scale, peak compensated admittance varies along the mmho scale), and often there is a region of possible scores for which a proportion of those with the disease overlaps with a proportion of those without the disease (Griner, Mayewski, Mashlin, & Greenland, 1981). Test criteria recommendations herein reflect a desire to find a test value that maximizes the performance of the test in identifying those with the disease while maintaining an acceptable rate of correctly identifying those without the disease.

To understand the screening process, it is necessary to understand how the performance of a screening test is estimated and how relevant variables interact. Also, the concepts of overlapping distributions and their relationship to sensitivity, specificity, prevalence, and predictive values need to be understood to evaluate test performance.

Sensitivity and Specificity

Sensitivity and specificity of a test relate to the ability of the test to identify correctly both those with the disease (sensitivity) and those without the disease (specificity). Sensitivity is the ratio of the number with the disease who are positive on the screening test to the number of all those with the disease. In other words, sensitivity represents the percentage labeled positive on the screening test of all those who truly have the target condition. Specificity is the ratio of the number of those without the disease who are negative on the screening test to the number of all those without the disease. In other words, specificity is the percentage labeled negative on the screening test of all those who truly are free of the target condition. To determine sensitivity and specificity, controlled clinical trials must be conducted. Screening results are compared to diagnostic test findings for verification of the patient's true status.

The overlapping distributions, and the resulting sensitivity and specificity, also provide information. That is, some individuals without the disease are referred for diagnosis and follow up (false-positive results) and some individuals with the disease are not referred (false-negative results). The false-positive rate (1 - specificity) and the false-negative rate (1 - sensitivity) depend on the degree of overlap of the two distributions on the continuum of test scores as well as the specific test criterion (i.e., cutoff) that is used.

Predictive Values

The test performance (sensitivity and specificity) together with the percentage of the population with the disease (disease prevalence) determine predictive values and the rates of over- and under-referral for diagnosis. Positive and negative predictive values are ratios also. Positive predictive value (PPV) is the ratio of the number of those scoring positive on the test who truly have the disease to the number of all those who scored positive on the test. Negative predictive value (NPV) is the ratio of the number of those scoring negative who truly do not have the disease to the number of all those scoring negative on the test. They are functions of sensitivity and specificity as well as the prevalence of the target condition. Whereas sensitivity and specificity of the test remain constant as long as the condition screened and the test criterion remain constant, predictive values vary with disease prevalence. In that regard, an estimate of prevalence of the condition must be known in addition to the sensitivity and specificity of the chosen test.

Over- and Under-Referral Rates

Predictive values determine over-referral and under-referral rates. The over-referral rate is the proportion of those referred who do not have the disease (1-PPV), and the under-referral rate is the proportion of those not referred who do have the disease (1-NPV). An unacceptably high over-referral rate can cause dissatisfaction among those being screened as well as those to whom the referrals are sent; it thereby reduces the effectiveness of the program. A high under-referral rate, which means that those with a disease are not identified, is also problematic and often results in delayed diagnosis and related consequences.

One mechanism for avoiding the problem of a high over-referral rate is to increase the prevalence of disease in the population screened. This is done by identifying a subgroup within the population that is at greater risk for having the target condition than the larger general population. Identification of a high-risk group can reduce an otherwise unmanageable over-referral rate to manageable proportions. Of course, there is a cost to such a decision. By selecting a high-risk subgroup for screening, those in the unscreened group who truly have the condition will be missed.

C. Screening Program Development and Management

The development of audiologic screening programs requires careful planning, implementation, and follow-up. Important program considerations include professional accountability and liability, risk management and quality improvement, and program evaluation.

Professional accountability and liability refer to the responsibility of the audiologist who develops, implements, and supervises the screening program to ensure appropriate patient care in all activities. These guidelines recommend that an audiologist be responsible for program accountability. Other personnel may perform the screening procedure (ASHA, 1981). Audiologists' responsibilities include developing mechanisms to ensure (a) patient confidentiality; (b) proper application of the screening protocol, including training and supervision of support personnel; and (c) appropriate patient counseling and referral.

These guidelines recommend obtaining informed consent, or, in the case of children, informed parental/legal guardian permission; however, extant state statutes or regulations, or institutional policies supersede this recommendation.

Risk management and quality assurance refer to the responsibility of the audiologist to evaluate risk factors associated with the screening program and to develop procedures to minimize or eliminate those factors. Risk factors in hearing screening programs may include potential for infection, inaccurate screening results based on equipment malfunction or errors in calibration, and errors in patient referral and follow-up. The audiologist is responsible for developing mechanisms to ensure (a) infection control through universal precautions (ASHA, 1991a; Ballachanda, Roeser, & Kemp, 1996; Joint Commission on Accreditation of Health Care Organizations, 1995; U.S. Department of Labor, Occupational Safety and Health Administration, 1991); (b) equipment calibration, electrical safety, and daily listening checks; and (c) accurate patient identification and recordkeeping. These quality assurance activities should include written documentation on a regular basis.

Program evaluation refers to the responsibility of the audiologist to evaluate the effectiveness of the screening program. This involves developing mechanisms to (a) quantify the pass and refer rates, (b) estimate the false-positive and false-negative rates, and (c) assure the effectiveness of follow-up protocols, especially for patients who are referred from the screening process. Program evaluation should occur on an ongoing basis to identify and correct factors that hinder optimum screening program performance and patient care.

The components of professional accountability and liability, risk management and quality assurance, and program evaluation must be developed prior to implementation of any screening program. Appropriate development of these components assists the audiologist in ensuring overall program quality and effectiveness.

D. Disorder, Impairment, and Disability

Consistent with terminology previously defined in the *Report on Audiologic Screening* (ASHA, 1995), the Panel developed separate guidelines for screening of hearing disorder, impairment, and disability. The Panel specifically adopted the following discrete definitions:

Disorder is any anatomic abnormality or pathology. It may or may not result in a change in function of a given organ or organ system.

Impairment is any loss or abnormality of psychological or physiological function. It implies that some functional aspect of an organ, system, or mechanism is outside a normal range.

Disability is any restriction or lack of ability to perform an activity by an individual (resulting from an impairment).

The Panel also considered the term *handicap* as defined by the ASHA Committee on Screening for Hearing Impairment, Handicap, and Middle Ear Disorders (ASHA, 1995).

Handicap is the difficulty experienced by an individual as a result of an impairment or disability and as a function of barriers (e.g., communication, structural, architectural, attitudinal), lack of accommodations, and/or lack of appropriate auxiliary aids and services (e.g., amplified telephone handset, assistive listening device) required for effective communication.

The Panel concluded that due to federal initiatives (Americans With Disabilities Act, Individuals With Disabilities Education Act) and consumer preferences (ASHA, 1994), the term *handicap* had undergone a process of definitional evolution. According to the World Health Organization definition (World Health Organization, 1980), the term *handicap* refers to a conflict between the person's performance or status and the expectations of his or her particular reference group.

As currently defined, persons with disabilities may find themselves in handicapping situations due to specific environmental restrictions or social expectations. The Panel concluded that it is inappropriate, therefore, to identify a person as having a hearing handicap. The Panel decided to refrain from employing the term *handicap* except in the "Screening for Auditory Disability" adult section, where it is used in reference to previous research and specific screening instruments.

E. Organizational Framework

The Panel adhered to a comprehensive organizational framework upon which separate sets of updated and new audiologic screening guidelines for disorder, impairment, and/or disability across age span could be drafted. Each set of guideline materials contains a general introductory section, an outline of recommended guidelines, and a discussion of important issues related to the assumptions and rationale underlying the Panel's recommendations.

The Panel asserts that all elements of each set should be fully considered prior to implementation of any guideline. The Panel's outlines of recommended guidelines are organized in a manner consistent with the *Preferred Practice Patterns for the Professions of Speech-Language Pathology and Audiology* document (ASHA, 1993); that is, recommendations include Personnel, Expected Outcome(s), Clinical Indications, Clinical Process, Pass/Refer Criteria, Setting/Equipment Specifications, and Documentation.

The present document accommodates two major sections, one for screening protocols for pediatric noninstitutionalized populations and one for screening protocols for adult noninstitutionalized populations. Each section contains introductory materials that reflect some special concerns regarding those populations. The pediatric section accommodates five sets of guidelines. One set pertains to screening infants and children for outer and middle ear disorder, and the remaining four sets (newborn, infant-toddlers, preschool, and school-age) address screening for impairment and disability.

The working group on screening adults developed three sets of guidelines: screening for disorder, screening for impairment, and screening for disability. Although each set is discrete, the panel strongly recommends that all three sets be implemented in adult audiologic screening programs.

These guidelines represent ASHA policy for audiologic screening practice, not standards. The Panel recognizes that each screening program and individual case represents unique characteristics that may influence the approach to screening program development and management and individual screening protocols. The Panel encourages audiologists to exercise professional judgment in the planning and implementation of screening programs.

F. References

American Speech-Language-Hearing Association. (1981, March). Guidelines for the employment and utilization of supportive personnel. *Asha, 23*, 165–169.

American Speech-Language-Hearing Association. (1985, May). Guidelines for identification audiometry. *Asha, 27*, 49–52.

American Speech-Language-Hearing Association. (1989, March). Audiologic screening of newborn infants who are at risk for hearing impairment. *Asha, 31*, 89–92.

American Speech-Language-Hearing Association. (1990, April). Guidelines for screening for hearing impairment and middle-ear disorders. *Asha, 32* (Suppl. 2), 17–24.

American Speech-Language-Hearing Association. (1991a). Chronic communicable diseases and risk management in the schools. *Language, Speech, and Hearing Services in Schools, 22*, 345–352.

American Speech-Language-Hearing Association. (1991b, March). Guidelines for the audiologic assessment of children from birth through 36 months of age. *Asha, 33* (Suppl. 5), 37–43.

American Speech-Language-Hearing Association. (1992, August). Report: Considerations in screening adults/older persons for handicapping hearing impairment. *Asha, 34*, 81–87.

American Speech-Language-Hearing Association. (1993). Preferred practice patterns for the professions of speech-language pathology and audiology. *Asha, 35* (Suppl. 11), 5–6.

American Speech-Language-Hearing Association. (1994, September). "Person first, please." *Asha, 36*, 10.

American Speech-Language-Hearing Association. (1995, February). Report on audiological screening. *American Journal of Audiology, 4*, 24–40.

Ballachanda, B. B., Roeser, R. J., & Kemp, R. J. (1996). Control and prevention of disease transmission in audiology practice. *American Journal of Audiology, 5* (1), 74–82.

Cadman, D., Chambers, L., Feldman, W., & Sackett, D. (1984). Assessing the effectiveness of community screening programs. *Journal of the American Medical Association, 252*, 1580–1585.

Feightner, J. W. (1992). Screening in the 1990's: Some principles and guidelines. In F. H. Bess & J. W. Hall III (Eds.), *Screening children for auditory function* (pp. 1–16). Nashville: Bill Wilkerson Center Press.

Frankenburg, W. K. (1974). Section of diseases and tests in pediatric screening. *Pediatrics, 54*, 612–616.

Griner, P. F., Mayewski, R. J., Mashlin, A. I., & Greenland, P. (1981). Selection and interpretation of diagnostic tests and procedures. *Annals of Internal Medicine, 92*, 557–570.

Hyde, M. L., Davidson, M. J., & Alberti, P. W. (1991). Auditory test strategy. In J. T. Jacobson & J. L. Northern (Eds.), *Diagnostic audiology*, 295–322. Austin, TX: Pro-Ed.

Joint Commission on Accreditation of Health Care Organizations. (1995). *Comprehensive accreditation manual for hospitals—Sect. 2, Surveillance, prevention, and control of infection*. Oakbrook Terrace, IL: JCAHO.

Joint Committee on Infant Hearing. (1994, December). Position Statement. *Asha, 36*, 38–41.

Swets, J. (1988). Measuring the accuracy of diagnostic systems. *Science, 240*, 1285–1293.

Thorner, R. M., & Remein, Q. R. (1982). Principles and procedures in the evaluation of screening for disease. In J. B. Chaiklin, I. M. Ventry, & R. F. Dixon (Eds.), *Hearing measurement: A book of readings* (2nd ed., pp. 408–421). Reading, MA: Addison-Wesley.

Turner, R. G. (1991). Making clinical decisions. In W. F. Rintelmann (Ed.), *Hearing assessment* (2nd ed., pp. 679–739). Austin, TX: Pro-Ed.

Turner, R. G. (1992a). Comparison of four hearing screening protocols. *Journal of the American Academy of Audiology, 3*, 200–207.

Turner, R. G. (1992b). Factors that determine the cost and performance of early identification protocols. *Journal of the American Academy of Audiology, 3*, 233–241.

Turner, R. G., & Cone-Wesson, B. (1992). Prevalence rates and cost-effectiveness of risk factors. In F. H. Bess & J. W. Hall III (Eds.), *Screening children for auditory function* (pp. 79–104). Nashville: Bill Wilkerson Center Press.

U.S. Department of Labor, Occupational Safety and Health Administration (1991, December 6). Occupational exposure to bloodborne pathogens: Final rule. Washington, DC: *Federal Register*.

Weinstein, M., & Fineberg, H. (1980). *Clinical decision making*. Philadelphia: Saunders.

World Health Organization (WHO). (1980). *International classification of impairments, disabilities, and handicaps: A manual of classification relating to consequences of disease* (pp. 25–43). World Health Organization.

II. Audiologic Screening Guidelines—Pediatric Section

The impact of childhood hearing impairment is well documented, particularly as it interferes with the development of speech and verbal language skills (Allen, 1986; Davis, 1988; Osberger, Moeller, Eccarius, Robbins, & Johnson, 1986; Osberger, Robbins, Lybolt, Kent, & Peters, 1986). Hearing impairment adversely affects the developing auditory nervous system and can have harmful effects on social, emotional, cognitive, and academic development, and, subsequently, on the individual's vocational and economic potential (Downs, 1994; Gravel, Wallace, & Ruben, 1995, 1996; National Institutes of Health, 1993).

The incidence of newborn hearing impairment is estimated to range from 1.5 to 6.0 per 1,000 live births (Parving, 1993; Watkin, Baldwin, & McEnery, 1991; White & Behrens, 1993). The prevalence rises in older infants and toddlers if mild conductive hearing losses associated with otitis media with effusion are included in the estimates. The most important period for language and speech development occurs during the first 3 years of life, but despite methods for identifying hearing impairment in newborns, the average age of identification in the United States continues to exceed 12 months (Harrison & Roush, 1996). Milder hearing impairments may go undetected even longer. It has become a national goal to reduce the age of identification to the first few months of life (Joint Committee on Infant Hearing, 1994; U.S. Department of Health and Human Services, Public Health Service, 1990).

Recent evidence indicates that the earlier impairment is identified and treatment begun, the greater the likelihood of preventing or reducing the debilitating/disabling effects that can result (Appuzo & Yoshinaga-Itano, 1995). Even children with unilateral hearing impairment remain at-risk for adverse academic and social-emotional effects (Bess, Klee, & Culbertson, 1986; Bess & Tharpe, 1986; Culbertson & Gilbert, 1986; Klee & Davis-Dansky, 1986; Oyler, Oyler, & Matkin, 1987, 1988). Children throughout the age range of birth through 18 years should receive hearing screening to detect congenital and/or acquired hearing impairment that may interfere with health, development, communication, and/or education.

A. Rationale

Although hearing disorder, impairment, and/or disability are prevalent among infants and children, a comprehensive set of screening guidelines for this population did not previously exist within a single document. This pediatric section contains audiologic screening guidelines that pertain to infants and children age birth through 18 years who have not been previously identified as having a hearing disorder, impairment, and/or disability, and to infants and children who can participate appropriately in the recommended process.

In the development of these audiologic screening guidelines, the Panel considered existing guidelines (ASHA, 1985, 1989, 1990, 1991, 1993). In these new guidelines that supersede previous ASHA screening guidelines, the Panel has attempted to synthesize current knowledge and to recommend appropriate clinical practice for children of all ages.

The Panel developed separate pediatric guidelines for hearing disorder and hearing impairment based on chronological age and developmental abilities:

1. Guidelines for screening for outer and middle ear disorder among older infants and children.

2. Guidelines for screening for hearing impairment among:

   • newborns and infants age birth through 6 months

   • infants and toddlers age 7 months through 2 years

   • preschool children age 3 to 5 years

   • school-age children age 5 through 18 years.

Children of all ages can receive reliable and valid screening for hearing impairment. For infants whose developmental age does not correspond with their chronological age (e.g., infants with developmental disabilities, infants who were born prematurely), the screening procedure selected should be appropriate to the child's developmental abilities.

Screening for hearing disability in children should be included in a general developmental screening of any child. In these sets of guidelines, screening for hearing disability is discussed below.

B. Personnel

Screening infants and children for hearing disorder and hearing impairment requires considerable professional expertise and technological sophistication. The Panel recommends that the screening process be designed, implemented, and supervised by an audiologist with the Certificate of Clinical Competence (CCC-A) from ASHA, and state licensure where applicable. Those cases where audiology support personnel may augment the audiologist's services are indicated in each guideline.

C. Informed Permission

These guidelines recommend obtaining informed parental/legal guardian permission; however, extant state statutes or regulations, or institutional policies, supersede this recommendation. Protocols should be developed that ensure patient confidentiality. The permission of the patient/legal guardian is the basic legal requisite necessary for disclosure of screening results to third parties (e.g., treatment programs or other professionals or agencies). The infant's or child's name should not be released without written permission of the parent(s) or guardian, the child's consent when he or she reaches the age of majority, or a court order (Andrews, 1985; Tharpe & Clayton, in press).

D. References

Allen, T. (1986). Patterns of academic achievement among hearing impaired students: 1974 and 1983. In A. Schildroth & M. Karchmer (Eds.) *Deaf children in America* (pp. 161–206). San Diego: College-Hill Press.

American Speech-Language-Hearing Association. (1985, May). Guidelines for identification audiometry. *Asha, 27*, 49–53.

American Speech-Language-Hearing Association. (1989, March). Audiologic screening of newborn infants who are at risk for hearing impairment. *Asha, 31*, 89–92.

American Speech-Language-Hearing Association. (1990, April). Guidelines for screening for hearing impairment and middle-ear disorders. *Asha, 32* (Suppl. 2), 17–24.

American Speech-Language-Hearing Association. (1991, March). Guidelines for the audiologic assessment of children from birth through 36 months of age. *Asha, 33* (Suppl. 5), 37–43.

American Speech-Language-Hearing Association. (1993, March). Preferred practice patterns for the professions of speech-language pathology and audiology. *Asha, 35* (Suppl. 11), 1–102.

Andrews, L. B. (Ed.) (1985). *Legal liability and quality assurance in newborn screening.* Chicago: American Bar Foundation.

Apuzzo, M. L. & Yoshinaga-Itano, C. (1995). Early identification of infants with significant hearing loss and the Minnesota Child Development Inventory. *Seminars in Hearing, 16*, 124–139.

Bess, F. H., Klee, T., & Culbertson, J. L. (1986). Identification, assessment, and management of children with unilateral sensorineural hearing loss. *Ear and Hearing, 7*, 43–51.

Bess, F. H. & Tharpe, A. M. (1986). Case history data on unilaterally hearing-impaired children. *Ear and Hearing, 7*, 14–19.

Culbertson, J., & Gilbert, L. (1986). Children with unilateral sensorineural hearing loss: Cognitive, academic, and social development. *Ear and Hearing, 7*, 38–42.

Davis, J. M. (1988). Management of the school age child: A psychosocial perspective. In F. Bess (Ed.), *Hearing impairment in children* (pp. 401–416). Parkton, MD: York Press.

Downs, M. P. (1994). The case for detection and intervention at birth. *Seminars in Hearing, 15*, 76–83.

Gravel, J. S., Wallace, I. F., & Ruben, R. J. (1995). Early otitis media and later educational risk. *Acta Otolaryngologica (Stockholm), 115*, 279–281.

Gravel, J. S., Wallace, I. F., & Ruben, R. J. (1996). Auditory consequences of early mild hearing loss associated with otitis media. *Acta Otolaryngologica (Stockholm), 116*, 219–221.

Harrison, M., & Roush, J. (1996). Age of suspicion, identification, and intervention for infants and young children with hearing loss: A national survey. *Ear and Hearing, 17*, 55–62.

Joint Committee on Infant Hearing. (1994). Position statement. *Asha, 36*, 38–41.

Klee, T., & Davis-Dansky, E. (1986). A comparison of unilaterally hearing-impaired children and normal-hearing children on a battery of standardized language tests. *Ear and Hearing, 7*, 27–37.

National Institutes of Health. (1993). *Early identification of hearing impairment in infants and young children: Consensus development conference.* Bethesda, MD: NIH.

Osberger M., Moeller, M., Eccarius, M., Robbins, A., & Johnson, D. (1986). Expressive language skills. In M. Osberger (Ed.), Language and learning skills in hearing impaired students. *ASHA Monographs, 23*, 54–65.

Osberger M., Robbins, A., Lybolt, J., Kent, R., & Peters, J. (1986). Speech evaluation. In M. Osberger (Ed.), Language and learning skills in hearing impaired students. *ASHA Monographs, 23*, 24–31.

Oyler, R. F., Oyler, A. L., & Matkin, N. D. (1987). Warning: A unilateral hearing loss may be detrimental to a child's academic career. *Hearing Journal, 40* (9), 18–22.

Oyler, R. F., Oyler, A. L., & Matkin, N. D. (1988). Unilateral hearing loss: Demographics and educational impact. *Language, Speech, and Hearing Services in Schools, 19*, 201–210.

Parving, A. (1993, May). Congenital hearing disability—Epidemiology and identification: A comparison between two health authority districts. *International Journal of Pediatric Otorhinolaryngology, 27* (1), 26–46.

Tharpe, A. M., & Clayton, E. W. (in press). Newborn hearing screening: Issues in legal liability and quality assurance. *American Journal of Audiology.*

U.S. Department of Health and Human Services, Public Health Service. (1990). *Healthy people 2000: National health promotion and disease prevention objectives.* Washington, DC: U.S. Government Printing Office.

Watkin, P. M., Baldwin, M., & McEnery, G. (1991, October). Neonatal at risk screening and the identification of deafness. *Archives of Disease in Childhood, 66* (10 Spec. No.), 1130–1135.

White, K. R., & Behrens, T. R. (Eds.) (1993). The Rhode Island Hearing Assessment Project: Implications for universal newborn hearing screening. *Seminars in Hearing, 14,* 1–122.

1. Guidelines for Screening Infants and Children for Outer and Middle Ear Disorders, Birth Through 18 Years

The issue of whether mass (universal) screening for middle ear disease is desirable or necessary continues to be debated (Bess, 1980; Bluestone et al., 1986; Lim, 1989; Lous, 1995; Northern, 1980; Task Force of the Symposium on Impedance Screening for Children, 1978) and must be resolved by the program administrator(s) based on circumstances specific to the goals of a given screening program. Many opposed to universal screening have argued that identification of high risk groups is a more cost effective and efficient means of identifying the majority of those who will have chronic middle ear disease. In that regard, no position on mass (universal) screening for middle ear disease is offered or implied in these guidelines.

The primary goal of outer and middle ear screening is to identify children with chronic otitis media with effusion (OME) that has the potential to cause significant medical problems, hearing loss, and/or long lasting speech, language, and learning deficits. However, the Panel is aware that many complex and controversial issues related to screening for middle ear disease remain unresolved (Bluestone et al., 1986). Some of the issues were debated by large groups of experts in 1977 (Bess, 1980; Northern, 1980; Task Force of the Symposium on Impedance Screening for Children, 1978) and again in 1984 (Bluestone et al., 1986). Concerns specifically related to screening for otitis media with effusion were addressed in the *Report of the Fourth Research Conference on Otitis Media* in 1987 (Lim, 1989).

The Panel concluded that identification of outer and middle ear disease is critical; it is a disease with high prevalence (U.S. Department of Health and Human Services, 1994) and high cost in terms of diagnosis and treatment, and has significant morbidity for a small percentage of those who have it. Despite the controversies and questions, there is general consensus that chronic middle ear disease in early childhood is a potentially significant disease that can have both medical and developmental consequences and that it should be identified and treated.

To screen children for outer and middle ear disorders, the Panel developed a single set of guidelines to apply across the pediatric age span. Screening for outer and middle ear disorders is essentially the same for all ages. It involves a pass/refer procedure to identify those children at risk for significant outer and middle ear disorders that have been undetected or untreated. The clinical process includes an optional case history, visual examination, and acoustic immittance testing.

Currently available instruments permit accurate detection of outer and middle ear disorders in the age range approximately 7 months through 18 years. Because the performance of acoustic immittance testing in identifying middle ear effusion (MEE) in young infants remains controversial, and access to that age group is limited to primary care physicians, the Panel refrained from developing guidelines that address screening for disorder in younger infants. In those cases, the Panel recommends that screening for outer and middle ear disorders be part of all well-baby examinations conducted by primary care practitioners (Lim, 1989).

Previously, ASHA (1979, 1990) produced two sets of guidelines related to screening for middle ear disorders. The original ASHA guidelines for screening for middle ear disorders (ASHA, 1979) included the acoustic immittance measures of tympanometry and the acoustic reflex. Unfortunately, that protocol resulted in high over-referral rates and was consequently rejected by professionals to whom children were referred, by parents and by school systems. In 1990, ASHA published a set of revised guidelines that were designed to (a) reduce the over-referral rate that accompanied the previous guidelines, (b) expand the scope of the screening beyond acoustic immittance alone, and (c) introduce a more objective quantitative, as opposed to the previous qualitative, approach to tympanogram interpretation. The Panel recognizes that since the 1990 guidelines were developed, relevant new knowledge and experience have become available.

The outline presented below contains the Panel's recommended guidelines for the development, supervision, and delivery of screening programs for outer and middle ear disorders in pediatric populations. The Panel provides a discussion of issues related to the rationale and assumptions underlying the recommendations. The Panel urges that this discussion section be considered fully prior to the implementation of the recommendations.

I. Personnel

Screening practitioners should be limited to:

A. Audiologists with Certificate of Clinical Competence (CCC-A) from the American Speech-Language-Hearing Association (ASHA) and state licensure where applicable (ASHA, 1996a).

B. Speech-language pathologists with Certificate of Clinical Competence (CCC-SLP) from the American Speech-Language-Hearing Association (ASHA) and state licensure where applicable (ASHA, 1996b).

C. Support personnel under supervision of a certified audiologist (ASHA, 1981).

II. Expected Outcomes

Identification of infants and children most likely to have:

A. Outer and middle ear conditions that may result in hearing loss or that may have significant health or developmental consequences.

B. Chronic or recurrent outer and middle ear disease.

III. Clinical Indications

A. Screen infants and children for outer and middle ear disorders as needed, requested, or mandated, or when they have conditions that place them at risk.

B. Screen infants and children from 7 months through 6 years of age. In the event that all of these children cannot be screened, it is recommended that children with the following characteristics be screened (Bluestone & Klein, 1996):

1. A first episode of acute otitis media prior to 6 months of age,

2. Infants who have been bottle fed,

3. Children with craniofacial anomalies, stigmata, or other findings associated with syndromes known to affect the outer and middle ear,

4. Ethnic populations with documented increased incidence of outer and middle ear disease (e.g., Native American and Eskimo populations),

5. A family history of chronic or recurrent OME,

6. Those in group day care settings and/or crowded living conditions,

7. Those exposed to excessive cigarette smoke, and

8. Children diagnosed with sensorineural hearing loss (Pappas, 1985), learning disabilities, behavior disorders, or developmental delays and disorders.

C. For children between 7 months and 6 years of age, screen for outer and middle ear disorders (Gates et al., 1989).

1. Conduct the first regularly scheduled screening program in the fall in conjunction with screening for hearing impairment (see age-appropriate guideline).

2. Conduct a second regularly scheduled screening program for those who failed or were missed in the fall.

D. Note that infants and children under the care of a physician for middle ear disorder need not participate in a screening program.

E. Note that infants and children not enrolled in organized child care programs, such as Head Start, should be screened for disorder at routine well-baby visits by primary care practitioners. (This type of screening is not within the scope of this document).

IV. Clinical Process

A. These guidelines recommend obtaining informed parental/legal guardian permission; however, extant state statutes or regulations, or institutional policies, supersede this recommendation.

B. Conduct screenings in a manner congruent with infection control and universal precautions (Ballachanda, Roeser, & Kemp, 1996; U.S. Department of Labor, Occupational Safety and Health Administration, 1991).

C. When possible, obtain a case history through verbal report of parent or guardian.

D. Visually inspect the ears to identify risk factors for outer and middle ear disease, and to ensure that no contraindications exist for performing tympanometry (e.g., drainage, foreign bodies, tympanostomy tubes).

E. As training and scope of practice (ASHA 1996b) permit, use a lighted otoscope or video-otoscope to examine the external ear canal and tympanic

Table 1. Equivalent ear canal volume measures for *children 1 to 7 years* of age prior to and following placement of tympanostomy tubes.[1]

90% range for ears with and without tubes	Pretube	Post-tube
Fifth percentile—95th percentile	0.3–0.9 cm³	1.0–5.5 cm³

[1] Shanks, Stelmachowicz, Beauchaine, and Schulte, 1992.

membrane (TM) for obvious obstructions or structural defects.

F. As training and scope of practice (ASHA 1996b) permit, perform tympanometry with a low frequency (220, 226 Hz) probe tone and a positive to negative air pressure sweep.

All hearing screening programs should include an educational component designed to provide parents with information, in lay language, on the process of ear disorder screening, the likelihood of their child having an ear disorder, and follow-up procedures.

V. Pass/Refer Criteria

A. Pass if no positive result exists for test criteria in both ears.

B. Refer for medical examination of the ears if:

1. ear drainage is observed.

2. visual identification of previously undetected structural defect(s) of ear occurs.

3. ear canal abnormalities such as obstructions, impacted cerumen or foreign objects, blood or other secretions, stenosis or atresia, otitis externa, and perforations or other abnormalities of the tympanic membrane are apparent.

4. tympanometric equivalent ear canal volume (V_{ec}) is greater than 1.0 cm³ accompanied by a flat tympanogram (i.e., there is no admittance peak) to select those at risk for TM perforation. Do not refer if tympanostomy tube is in place or a perforation of the TM is under management of a physician. See Table 1 for estimates of a normal range for V_{ec}, assuming compensation for ear canal volume at +200 daPa.

5. follow-up tympanometric screening (i.e., rescreen) test results are outside the test criteria presented in Table 2. Because prevalence of middle ear disorders in the group referred for rescreening is often greater than in the group screened initially, screening program administrators may consider modifying pass/refer criteria to optimize program performance (see discussion).

Table 2. Recommended initial tympanometric screening test criteria.

Infants[a]	One year to school age[b]
Y_{tm}<0.2 mmho or TW>235 daPa	Y_{tm}<0.3 mmho[1] or TW>200 daPa

Legend: mmho = millimho; daPa = decaPascal; TW = tympanometric width; Y_{tm} = peak admittance

[a] Infants: Roush, Bryant, Mundy, Zeisel, and Roberts, 1995

[b] Older Children: Nozza, Bluestone, Kardatzke, and Bachman, 1992; 1994

[1] For children >6 years of age, when using ±400 daPa for compensation of ear canal volume, Y_{tm}<0.4 mmho is the recommended criterion.

C. Refer for rescreening if:

 1. initial tympanometric screening test results are outside test cutoffs as presented in Table 2.

D. Be aware that the recommended test criteria may need to be adjusted based on important factors specific to each individual program (See Discussion).

E. Note that pathologies that increase admittance of the middle ear (e.g., ossicular discontinuity) will not be identified.

VI. Inappropriate Procedures

A. The following are not recommended:

 1. pure-tone hearing screening to identify those at risk for outer or middle ear disease;

 2. otoscopic examination alone for identification of those at risk for outer or middle ear disease;

 3. acoustic reflectometry;

 4. tympanometric peak pressure (TPP);

 5. acoustic reflex tests; and

 6. otoacoustic emissions screening measures.

VII. Follow-Up Procedures

Based on review of the supervising audiologist, the following recommendations may be made:

A. Recommend immediate medical evaluation for child referred due to:

 1. case history (if completed), visual inspection or otoscopic screening results demonstrating otalgia or otorrhea; and

 2. tympanometric equivalent ear canal volume (V_{ec}) and flat tympanogram results indicating TM perforation(s).

B. Rescreen child referred based on criteria in Table 2 within 6 to 8 weeks from the time of the initial test.

C. Recommend immediate medical evaluation for the child when rescreening results continue to indicate an abnormality.

D. Communicate promptly with parents or other caretakers and make a medical referral to, in most cases, the family physician.

E. Request information regarding the outcome of follow-up audiological evaluations or medical examinations. The supervising audiologist should monitor, and may participate in, the management of the child.

VIII. Setting/Equipment Specifications

A. Screen in an environment conducive to tympanometry and lighted otoscopy.

B. Use a lighted otoscope or video-otoscope.

C. Use a screening or diagnostic tympanometer. Note that some instruments are restricted for certain test parameters, so the influence of different instrumentation settings on tympanometric measures must be considered.

D. Meet American National Standards Institute specifications for instruments to measure aural acoustic impedance and admittance (aural acoustic immittance) (ANSI S3.39-1987).

E. Meet manufacturer's specification for calibration and regulatory agency specification of equipment for electrical safety.

IX. Documentation

A. Record identifying information, screening/rescreening results, and recommended follow-up procedures. Include names of personnel conducting the screening/rescreening.

B. Record case history (if completed), otoscopic and tympanometric results.

C. Document follow-up results and personnel conducting follow-up.

Discussion

Epidemiological studies indicate that prevalence of MEE increases through the winter months; thus, one might argue for screening during that time of the year. However, a high percentage of the cases of OME during the winter are associated with upper respiratory tract infections (URI). The need to aggressively seek out such episodes of OME is small because children with URI often receive medical attention, and OME associated with URI often resolves with resolution of the URI (Gates et al., 1989). Some underserved populations, however, may not get medical attention promptly even for URI, so screening during seasons of high incidence and prevalence is indicated.

It is not cost effective to screen the general population of children 7 years of age and older because the potential yield is very low (Lous, 1995; Gates et al., 1989). However, some groups of children are at increased risk for OME or are especially vulnerable to effects of auditory disorders. Individual program administrators may choose to screen such children after they are 7 years of age. Populations considered to be at greater risk for OME include those of certain ethnic backgrounds such as Native American and Eskimo, those who live in crowded conditions, those with craniofacial anomalies, stigmata, or other findings or syndromes associated with otitis media with effusion, and possibly those exposed to cigarette smoke in the home. In addition, children with sensorineural hearing impairment, learning disabilities, and other conditions that might affect learning should continue to be screened for middle ear disorders throughout the school years.

Clinical Process

In the previous Guidelines (ASHA, 1990), case history and visual inspection were recommended as possible ways to reduce over-referrals that result from tympanometric screening. Despite the paucity of data on the efficacy of case history and/or screening by visual examination, this Panel recommends also that screening programs include such measures. Programs that develop mechanisms for screening using case history and/or visual examination are encouraged to collect and share information on efficacy of these measures.

Pass/Refer Criteria

Tympanometric equivalent ear canal volume (V_{ec}) outside the normal range accompanied by a tympanogram with no peak may indicate an opening in the TM. Unless a child has a tympanotomy tube in place or is known to have a TM perforation that is under management of a physician, an immediate referral for medical examination is indicated.

Tympanometric criteria for referral when screening for MEE vary depending on factors related to the population screened, such as age and prevalence of middle ear disease, as well as resources for follow-up and factors related to instrumentation settings. Factors related to the population, the test parameters, the disease as defined by the screening program administrators, and the availability of diagnostic referral resources also affect the choice of a referral criterion (Nozza, 1995).

Tympanometric peak pressure (TPP) is not included in the criteria for identifying children at risk for OME. TPP was excluded from the guidelines developed by ASHA in 1990. It was stated that "...negative TPP associated with an otherwise normal tympanogram is a poor determinant of middle ear effusion. Furthermore, abnormal TPP in the absence of other tympanic membrane abnormalities does not reflect a change in the mechanical properties of the middle ear..." Wiley and Smith (1995) in reviewing TPP in screening report that "...its use in middle ear screening results in poor specificity or high false positive rates." New data on performance of tympanometric variables for identifying MEE have been reported (Nozza et al., 1992; 1994, Silman, Silverman, & Arick, 1992). Although Silman et al. (1992) recommend test criteria that include TPP, Nozza et al. (1992, 1994) found TPP to be of little value in identifying ears with middle ear effusion.

In the absence of data, an alternative method based on the limits of the normal range may be used to determine screening test criteria. For infants above 7 months with normal middle ear function, the 5th percentile for peak compensated static acoustic admittance (Y_{tm}) is 0.2 mmho, so one choice for a test criterion would be <0.2 mmho (Roush et al., 1995). In that case, specificity is set to 95% because only 5% of normal ears would be below the cutoff value. In a similar way, tympanometric width (TW)>235 daPa would have 95% specificity because 235 daPa is at the 95th percentile of normal ears (Roush et al., 1995). However, when using data from normal ears to select a screening criterion, information on the distribution of test scores for abnormal ears is lacking, so no estimate of sensitivity can be made. A screening program that relies on criteria determined using only normative data must monitor program performance carefully and use information on program outcomes to modify screening test criteria, if necessary.

For infants and children from 1 year to school age, Y_{tm}<0.3 mmho or TW>200 daPa are recommended screening criteria. These values have been shown to be just outside the normal range for infants under 30 months (Roush et al., 1995) and also have been shown to have high specificity and good sensitivity in children of school age (Nozza, 1995; Nozza et al., 1994; Silman, Silverman, & Arick, 1992, 1994). These values are slightly different from those reported in the 1990 ASHA guidelines [i.e., Y_{tm}<0.2 mmho or TW>150 daPa], which were based on normative data from children 4 to 6 years of age. The new recommended cutoffs should produce greater specificity with only negligible adverse effects on sensitivity in screening programs that address unselected groups of children in the general population such as might attend pre-schools or elementary schools. In a low prevalence disease that has nonlethal sequelae and for which over-referrals can be a problem, maximizing specificity is considered desirable (Gates et al., 1989).

It has been shown that in a very high-risk group of children, that is, with a history of chronic MEE and scheduled for myringotomy and tube surgery, the criteria Y_{tm}<0.2 or TW>300 have high sensitivity and specificity (Nozza et al., 1994). Obviously, the children undergoing surgery are the extreme cases in terms of OME severity. For groups of children who are at greater risk than the general population but who do not meet criteria for myringotomy and tube surgery, a slightly different criterion might serve better. As stated above, by monitoring screening program outcomes, program administrators can adjust test criteria to reach satisfactory pass and refer rates.

The recommended criteria offered in this document are considered to be first approximations for the situations described. The recommended criteria for infants 6 to 12 months of age are based on limited data. For older children, there are more complete data. The cutoffs of $Y_{tm}<0.3$ mmho or TW>200 daPa should serve well for programs involving children from the general population. For programs with children at greater risk for chronic or recurrent OME, that is, with higher prevalence of OME and/or more severe cases, different criteria might be necessary to keep over-referral rates to manageable proportions.

Follow-Up Procedures

This guideline recommends that a child with unilateral or bilateral tympanogram meeting referral criteria other than those that are consistent with a TM perforation should be rescreened 6 to 8 weeks after the initial test. Because middle ear disease is often self-limiting, referral based on a single screening is generally not recommended. Various schemes for a two-screening protocol have been suggested (see ASHA, 1979; Lous, 1983; Northern, 1992; Roush, 1990 for additional information on retest criteria). Most suggested screen-rescreen protocols attempt on the first screening to identify a group at risk from the general population being screened. Then the rescreening, usually at about 6 or 8 weeks following the initial screening, is administered to further separate those with a high probability of chronic middle ear disease from those with transient disease. The screening criteria recommended above for infants and children in the general population are based on an assumption that the initial screening is of a group of children for whom the prevalence of middle ear disease is fairly low. The initial screening pass/refer criteria are designed to have high sensitivity with the understanding that specificity might be low; that is, on retest there will probably be many who will pass.

Inappropriate Procedures

Pure-tone hearing screening to identify those at risk for outer or middle ear disease is not recommended. There are no data available that report reasonable specificity for a hearing screening for identification of those at risk for middle ear disease. Silman, Silverman, and Arick (1994) and Silverman (1995) have reported recently that hearing impairment screening had good sensitivity for identification of ears with MEE. However, they report no specificity

data, so the Panel does not feel that this information can be used to justify a change in the screening protocol recommendation at this time.

Otoscopic inspection alone for identification of those at risk for middle ear disease is not recommended. Identification of MEE using an otoscope requires training and skill beyond that available to most programs designed to screen for middle ear disease. The visual inspection component of the screening guidelines is not intended to suggest that pass/refer decisions be made based on identification of middle ear disease. Rather, the intent is to use visual inspection as a means to identify gross abnormalities of the outer ear that would require immediate medical examination.

Acoustic reflectometry has not proven to have sufficient performance characteristics (sensitivity, specificity, and predictive ability) to be recommended for use in screening protocols. Whereas the potential for this instrument to provide an easy and quick screening for middle ear disease has been reported, research has not demonstrated efficacy of that procedure. At the time of this writing, there is no commercially available instrument for acoustic reflectometry testing for purposes of clinical assessment or screening.

The acoustic reflex test is associated with a high probability of false-positive identifications and questionable validity, especially when using automated instruments such as those used in many large screening programs. Failure to elicit an acoustic reflex is considered a positive result when the acoustic reflex is used in screening for middle ear disorder. To consider the absence of the acoustic reflex as positive assumes auditory function sufficient to produce an acoustic reflex in the absence of middle ear disease and integrity of all of the components of a reflex arc involving the cranial nerves VII and VIII. Some researchers have reported good performance of the acoustic reflex, under specific test conditions and population characteristics, and have suggested further research in that area (e.g., Silman & Emmer, 1995; Silman, Silverman, & Arick, 1992). However, the false positive rates reported for screening with the acoustic reflex have consistently been high (Lous, 1983; Nozza et al., 1992; Roush & Tait, 1985). Also, children with sensorineural hearing impairment and those with possible neurological problems that may interfere with the acoustic reflex arc must be screened also, but they would not be eligible for a screening that includes the acoustic reflex. That is, a screening test that is more directly related to the function being screened is favored. The acoustic reflex test is not recommended for screening for middle ear disorders.

Otoacoustic emissions testing holds promise for screening young children for hearing loss. It has also been suggested that such testing might be useful for identifying those at risk for middle ear disorders as well (Decreton, Hanssens, & DeSlooveres, 1991; Nozza & Sabo, 1992). However, there are too few data available regarding this test for screening infants and children to demonstrate efficacy at this time.

Setting/Equipment Specifications

Either a screening or diagnostic tympanometer may be used. Some instruments are restricted for certain test parameters, so the influence of different instrumentation parameters on tympanometric measures must be considered. It is also important to remember that values such as Y_{tm} are influenced by instrumentation settings. Most notably, the air pressure used for compensation of ear canal volume and the rate of pressure sweep can both affect the tympanometric data. The recommended criteria are based on data from different studies that have used different instrumentation settings (ASHA, 1990; Nozza et al., 1994). Program administrators responsible for setting protocols should be aware of the data on test performance and how the data were obtained.

References

American National Standards Institute. (1987). *American national standard specifications for instruments to measure aural acoustic impedance and admittance (aural acoustic immittance)*. ANSI S3.39. New York: ANSI.

American Speech-Language-Hearing Association. (1979). Guidelines for acoustic immittance screening of middle ear function. *Asha, 21,* 283–288.

American Speech-Language-Hearing Association. (1981). Guidelines for the employment and utilization of supportive personnel. *Asha, 23,* 165–169.

American Speech-Language-Hearing Association. (1990, April). Guidelines for screening for hearing impairments and middle ear disorders. *Asha, 32* (Suppl. 2), 17–24.

American Speech-Language-Hearing Association. (1996a, Spring). Scope of practice in audiology. *Asha, 38* (Suppl. 16), 12–15.

American Speech-Language-Hearing Association. (1996b, Spring). Scope of practice in speech-language pathology. *Asha, 38* (Suppl. 16), 1–4.

Ballachanda, B. B., Roeser, R. J., & Kemp, R. J. (1996). Control and prevention of disease transmission in audiology practice. *American Journal of Audiology, 5* (1), 74–82.

Bess, F. H. (1980). Impedance screening for children: A need for more research. *Annals of Otology, Rhinology, and Laryngology, 89* (Suppl. 68), 228–232.

Bluestone, C. D., Fria, T. J., Arjona, S. K., Casselbrant, M. L., Schwartz, D. M., Ruben, R. J., Gates, G. A., Downs, M. P., Northern, J. L., Jerger, J. F., Paradise, J. L., Bess, F. H., Kenworthy, O. T., & Rogers, K. D. (1986). Controversies in screening for middle ear disease and hearing loss in children. *Pediatrics, 77,* 57–70.

Bluestone, C. D., & Klein, J. O. (1996). Otitis media, atelectasis, and eustachian tube disfunction. In C. D. Bluestone, S. E. Stool, & M. A. Kenna (Eds.), *Pediatric Otolaryngology* (3rd ed., vol. I, pp. 388–582). Philadelphia: Saunders.

Decreton, S. J. R. C., Hanssens, K., & DeSloovere, M. (1991). Evoked otoacoustic emissions in infant hearing screening. *International Journal of Pediatric Otorhinolaryngology, 21,* 235–247.

Gates, A. G., Northern, J. L., Ferrer, H. P., Jerger, J., Marchant, C. D., Fiellau-Nikolajsen, M., Ranney, J. B., Renvall, U., Ruben, R. J., Stewart, I., & Teele, D. W. . (1989, April). Diagnosis and screening. In D. J. Lim (Ed.), Recent advances in otitis media: Report of the Fourth Research Conference. *Annals of Otology, Rhinology, and Laryngology, 98* (Suppl. 139), 4, Part 2.

Lim, D. J. (Ed.). (1989). Recent advances in otitis media: Report of the Fourth Research Conference. *Annals of Otology, Rhinology, and Laryngology, 98* (Suppl. 139), 4, 2.

Lous, J. (1983). Three impedance screening programs on a cohort of seven-year-old children. *Scandinavian Audiology,* (Suppl. 17), 60–64.

Lous, J. (1995). Secretory otitis media in schoolchildren: Is screening for secretory otitis media advisable? *Danish Medical Bulletin, 42* (1), 71–99.

Northern, J. L. (1980). Impedance screening: An integral part of hearing screening. *Annals of Otology, Rhinology, and Laryngology, 89* (Suppl. 68), 233–235.

Northern, J. L. (1992). Special issues concerned with screening for middle ear disease in children. In F. H. Bess & J. W. Hall III (Eds.), *Screening children for auditory function* (pp. 39–60). Nashville: Bill Wilkerson Center Press.

Nozza, R. J. (1995). Critical issues in acoustic-immittance screening for middle-ear effusion. *Seminars in Hearing, 16* (1), 86–98.

Nozza, R. J., Bluestone, C. D., Kardatzke, D., & Bachman, R. N. (1992). Toward the validation of aural acoustic immittance measures for diagnosis of middle ear effusion in children. *Ear and Hearing, 13* (6), 442–453.

Nozza, R. J., Bluestone, C. D., Kardatzke, D., & Bachman, R. N. (1994). Identification of middle ear effusion by aural acoustic admittance and otoscopy. *Ear and Hearing, 15,* 310–323.

Nozza, R. J., & Sabo, D. L. (1992). Transient evoked OAE for screening school-age children. *Hearing Journal, 45* (11), 29–31.

Pappas, D. G. (1985). *Diagnosis and treatment of hearing impairment in children*. San Diego: College-Hill Press.

Roush, J. (1990). Identification of hearing loss and middle ear disease in preschool and school-age children. *Seminars in Hearing, 11* (4), 357–371.

Roush, J., Bryant, K., Mundy, M., Zeisel, S., & Roberts, J. (1995). Developmental changes in static admittance and tympanometric width in infants and toddlers. *Journal of the American Academy of Audiology, 6,* 334–338.

Roush, J., & Tait, C. (1985). Pure tone and acoustic immittance screening of pre-school-age children: An examination of referral criteria. *Ear and Hearing, 6* (5), 245–249.

Shanks, J. E., Stelmachowicz, P. G., Beauchaine, K. L., & Schulte, L. (1992). Equivalent ear canal volumes in children pre- and post-tympanostomy tube insertion. *Journal of Speech and Hearing Research, 35,* 936–941.

Silman, S., & Emmer, M. B. (1995). Ipsilateral acoustic reflex in middle ear effusion. In S. Silman & M. B. Emmer (Eds.), Audiologic and medical profiles of middle-ear effusion. *Seminars in Hearing, 19* (1), 80–85.

Silman, S., Silverman, C. A., & Arick, D. S. (1992). Acoustic-immittance screening for detection of middle-ear effusion in children. *Journal of the American Academy of Audiology, 3,* 262–268.

Silman, S., Silverman, C. A., & Arick, D. S. (1994). Pure-tone assessment and screening of children with middle-ear effusion. *Journal of the American Academy of Audiology, 5,* 173–182.

Silverman, C. A. (1995). Pure tone characteristics of children with middle-ear effusion. In S. Silman & M. B. Emmer (Eds.), Audiologic and medical profiles of middle-ear effusion, *Seminars in Hearing, 19* (1), 99–104.

Task Force of the Symposium on Impedance Screening for Children. (1978). Use of acoustic impedance measurement in screening for middle ear disease in children. *Pediatrics, 62,* 570–573.

U.S. Department of Health and Human Services. (1994). *Otitis media with effusion in young children* (Clinical Practice Guideline, No. 12). AHCPR Pub. No. 94-0622. Rockville, MD: Agency for Health Care Policy and Research, HHS.

U.S. Department of Labor, Occupational Safety and Health Administration. (1991, December 6). Occupational exposure to bloodborne pathogens: Final rule. Washington, DC: *Federal Register.*

Wiley, T. L., & Smith, P. S. U. (1995). Acoustic-immittance measures and middle-ear screening. *Seminars in Hearing, 16* (1), 60–79.

2. Guidelines for Screening for Hearing Impairment— Neonates and Young Infants, Birth Through 6 Months

Carefully designed and implemented screening programs improve early identification of babies with hearing impairment (White et al., 1994). As recognized by the U.S. Department of Health and Human Services, Public Health Service (1990), the National Institutes of Health Consensus Panel (1993), and the Joint Committee on Infant Hearing (1994), early identification of and intervention for childhood hearing impairment is a national health objective.

In 1994, the Joint Committee on Infant Hearing endorsed the goal of universal detection of infants with hearing impairment as early as possible (Joint Committee on Infant Hearing, 1994). The Joint Committee specified that all infants with hearing impairment should be identified before 3 months of age and receive intervention by 6 months of age. To achieve this goal, screening all newborn infants with physiologic auditory measures is recommended to identify those infants most likely to have peripheral hearing impairment that may interfere with health, development, communication, or education. For infants not screened at birth, these guidelines may be applied for infants through developmental age approximately 6 months.

Hearing impairment is defined as unilateral or bilateral sensorineural and/or conductive hearing levels of greater than 20 dB HL. Current screening methodologies for this population allow reliable detection of hearing impairments of greater than 30 dB HL. Screening for unilateral hearing impairment is recommended to identify infants and young children at risk for communicative and academic difficulties (Bess, Klee, & Culbertson, 1986; Bess & Tharpe, 1986; Culbertson & Gilbert, 1986; Klee & Davis-Dansky, 1986; Oyler, Oyler, & Matkin, 1987, 1988). Because behavioral screening procedures do not yield accurate predictions of hearing impairment for neonates and very young infants (Durieux-Smith, Picton, Bernard, MacMurray, & Goodman, 1991; Joint Committee on Infant Hearing, 1994), the presence of hearing impairment may be inferred from physiologic measures (auditory brainstem response and/or otoacoustic emissions). In these cases, estimates may correlate well with hearing sensitivity in a limited range of frequencies.

The following outline contains recommended guidelines for the development, supervision, and delivery of screening programs for hearing impairment in neonates and infants (birth through 6 months of age). The Panel provides a discussion of issues related to the rationale and assumptions underlying its recommendations. The Panel intends that this discussion section be fully considered prior to implementation of the recommendations.

I. Personnel

Limit screening practitioners to:

A. Audiologists with Certificate of Clinical Competence (CCC-A) from the American Speech-Language-Hearing Association (ASHA) and state licensure where applicable (ASHA, 1996).

B. Support personnel under supervision of a certified audiologist (ASHA, 1981).

II. Expected Outcome

Identification of newborns and young infants at risk for hearing impairment that may affect health, communication, and development.

III. Clinical Indications

A. Screen all newborn infants with physiologic auditory measures that correlate with hearing sensitivity.

B. If all newborn infants cannot be screened due to resource limitations or other considerations, screen all infants who receive neonatal intensive or special care (Davis, Wood, Healy, Webb, & Rowe, 1995; Mauk, White, Mortensen, & Behrens, 1991), and all infants who have conditions that place them at risk (with indicators) for hearing impairment. Associated indicators include (Joint Committee on Infant Hearing, 1994):

1. family history of hereditary childhood sensorineural hearing loss,

2. in utero infection, such as cytomegalovirus, rubella, syphilis, herpes, and toxoplasmosis,

3. craniofacial anomalies, including those with morphological abnormalities of the pinna and ear canal,

4. birth weight less than 1,500 grams (3.3 lbs),

5. hyperbilirubinemia at a serum level requiring exchange transfusion,

6. ototoxic medications, including but not limited to the aminoglycosides, used in multiple courses or in combination with loop diuretics,

7. bacterial meningitis,

8. Apgar scores of 0–4 at 1 minute or 0–6 at 5 minutes,

9. mechanical ventilation lasting 5 days or longer,

10. stigmata or other findings associated with a syndrome known to include sensorineural and/or conductive hearing loss,

11. parent/caregiver concern regarding hearing and/or developmental delay,

12. head trauma associated with loss of consciousness or skull fracture,

13. recurrent or persistent otitis media with effusion for at least 3 months.

C. For infants born in hospitals, screening should be done as close to hospital discharge as possible (Kok, vanZanten, Brocaar, & Wallenburg, 1993).

D. Children may pass an initial hearing screening but be at risk for fluctuating, delayed-onset, or progressive sensorineural and/or conductive hearing impairment. Those children's hearing should be monitored at least every 6 months until 3 years of age, and at intervals thereafter dependent on the risk factors (Joint Committee on Infant Hearing, 1994). Risk conditions include:

1. family history of hereditary childhood hearing loss,

2. in utero infection such as cytomegalovirus, rubella, syphilis, herpes, or toxoplasmosis,

3. neurofibromatosis type II and neurodegenerative disorders,

4. recurrent or persistent otitis media with effusion,

5. anatomic deformities and other disorders that affect eustachian tube function.

III. Clinical Process

A. These guidelines recommend obtaining informed parental/legal guardian permission; however, extant state statutes or regulations, or institutional policies, supersede this recommendation.

B. Conduct screening in a manner congruent with infection control and universal precautions (Ballachanda, Roeser, & Kemp, 1996; U.S. Department of Labor, Occupational Safety and Health Administration, 1991).

C. Screen for hearing impairment using one or two recommended physiologic measures. The auditory brainstem response (ABR) is a physiologic measure of peripheral auditory function through the brainstem. The evoked otoacoustic emission (EOAE) is a physiologic measure of preneural auditory function. The choice of screening measure may influence program outcome. (See discussion.) Both physiologic measures should be obtained while the infant is in a quiet or sleeping state. The recommended procedures are:

1. ABR:

a) Either operator-controlled or automated ABR (Jacobson, Jacobson, & Spahr, 1990; Kennedy et al., 1991);

b) Note that recommended stimulus conditions include presentation of air-conducted click stimuli to each ear at 35 dB nHL or lower, with a stimulus rate upper limit of 37/second (Jacobson & Hall, 1994);

c) Alternating polarity may be appropriate in screening applications when presence or absence of wave V is the only criteria used to determine a pass/refer outcome;

d) For automated ABR, number of repetitions will be determined automatically by manufacturer protocol. For operator-controlled ABR, a minimum of 1,000 repetitions is required under optimal recording conditions to yield reliable screening results (Hall, 1992). In less optimal recording conditions (e.g., excessive noise or physiologic artifact), more repetitions may be required;

e) Wave V amplitude is enhanced in the neonate when a high-pass filter of 30 Hz is used (Hall, Brown, & Mackay-Hargadine, 1985; Sininger, 1995; Stuart & Yang, 1994) and if an electrode montage of Fz-nape of neck rather than Fz-ipsilateral ear configuration is used (Katabamna, Bennett, Dokler, & Metz, 1995;

Sininger, Cone-Wesson, & Ma, 1994; Sininger, 1993).

2. otoacoustic emissions (OAE) (Joint Committee on Infant Hearing, 1994; National Institutes of Health, 1993).

a) Otoacoustic emission screening protocols vary. Either transient evoked (TEOAE) or distortion product otoacoustic emissions (DPOAE) may be appropriate for neonatal screening (Bergman, Gorga, Neely, Kaminski, Beauchaine, & Peters, 1995);

b) For TEOAE, the suggested stimulus conditions are: broad-band clicks presented at 50–80/second at 80 dB pe SPL (Maxon, White, Mortensen, & Behrens, 1995);

c) For DPOAE, the suggested stimulus conditions are: f2/f1=1.2, with f2 at 2, 3, and 4 KHz; L2 = 55 dB SPL; L1 = 65 dB SPL (Gaskill & Brown, 1990; Harris, Lonsbury-Martin, Stagner, Coats, & Martin, 1989; Stover, Gorga, Neely, & Montoya, 1996);

d) Remove probe if response is not seen, and inspect for debris before reinserting. Alternately, the probe should be removed and visual inspection with an otoscope should be performed before reinserting the probe (Vohr, White, & Maxon, 1996).

D. All hearing screening programs should include an educational component designed to provide parents with information, in lay language, on the process of hearing screening, the likelihood of their child having a hearing impairment, and follow-up procedures. Parent education regarding normal auditory, speech, and language development should also be included in the hearing screening program.

V. Pass/Refer Criteria

A. Pass if reliable responses are present at the screening criterion for both ears.

1. ABR pass if reliable evoked responses are present at 35 dB nHL or lower (Hyde, Riko, & Malizia, 1990; Durieux-Smith et al, 1991).

2. EOAE pass if an acceptable signal-to-noise (S/N) ratio or reproducibility are reached. Firm criteria for S/N and reproducibility are not yet established. It is important to recognize that percent reproducibility and S/N are not independent measurements (Gorga et al., 1993a; 1993b).

B. Refer if a reliable response is absent at the screening criterion from either ear.

VI. Acceptable Modifications

A. Assimilate, as appropriate, new technologies or improvements to existing technologies (e.g., automated recordkeeping, noise detection and reduction) that substantially enhance infant hearing screening (Joint Committee on Infant Hearing, 1994).

VII. Inappropriate Procedures

Do not use behavioral measures, including automated behavioral techniques, to screen newborns and very young infants. These procedures cannot validly and reliably detect mild hearing impairment in newborns (Durieux-Smith, Picton, Edwards, Goodman, & MacMurray, 1985) and very young infants (Joint Committee on Infant Hearing, 1994).

VIII. Follow-Up Procedures

A. Recommend that an infant who is referred from screening receive either (a) rescreening (ABR or OAE) (National Institutes of Health, 1993; White, Vohr, & Behrens, 1993), or (b) audiologic evaluation, including threshold ABR measures that may be completed immediately following the initial or follow-up screening (Galambos, Wilson, & Silva, 1994; Stein, Ozdamar, Kraus, & Paton, 1983).

B. For infants referred from screening, confirm auditory status optimally within 1 month but no later than 3 months after the initial screening.

IX. Setting/Equipment Specifications

A. Conduct screening in an environment where ambient noise levels are sufficiently low to permit reliable measurements.

1. Infant's activity level may affect the outcome of ABR screening (McCall & Ferraro, 1991), and electrical interference in the NICU may complicate accurate ABR screening.

2. High ambient noise levels, typically greater than 60 dBA, have been reported in neonatal intensive care units (NICU) (Mitchell, 1984). Whenever possible, efforts should be made to test in quiet locations.

3. Ambient room noise and the physiologic noise of the infants are two primary noise sources during EOAE screening.

4. Background noise level should not exceed 55 dBA during OAE screening (Kemp & Ryan, 1993). A quiet and sleeping infant enhances the likelihood of a reliable and valid response

(Vohr, White, Maxon, & Johnson, 1993) as does a good probe fit (Kemp, Ryan, & Bray, 1990).

B. Meet manufacturers' specification for calibration and regulatory agency specification for electrical safety of all equipment.

X. Documentation

A. Document identifying information, screening results, and recommendations for follow-up procedures.

B. Request parent's or legal guardian's permission to obtain results of follow-up procedures.

C. If possible, document follow-up results and personnel conducting follow-up.

Discussion

Screening the hearing of newborns and very young infants has been advocated for decades (Downs, 1967; Galambos & Hecox, 1978; Hosford-Dunn, Johnson, Simmons, Malachowski, & Low, 1987; Joint Committee on Infant Hearing, 1994; National Institutes of Health, 1993). In development and implementation of newborn/very young infant hearing screening programs, audiologists should consider several unresolved issues. Those issues include the limitations of physiologic test procedures for predicting hearing sensitivity, test performance characteristics of the recommended screening procedures, and the impact of false-negative and false-positive screening results.

Clinical Process

Physiologic procedures do not provide a direct measure of hearing sensitivity. Rather, physiologic procedures provide a direct measure of a physiologic process that may correlate with hearing sensitivity. It has been demonstrated in older children and adults, for example, that the ABR provides a direct measure of neural transmission in the eighth nerve and pontine-level auditory pathway, and correlates with behavioral hearing measures in the mid- to-high frequency region. OAEs provide a direct estimate of outer hair cell integrity and cochlear function, which yields an indirect estimate of peripheral hearing sensitivity. Both click-evoked ABR and OAEs yield best estimates of high-frequency (e.g., 2–4KHz) sensitivity (Coats & Martin, 1977; Gorga et al., 1993a, 1993b; Gorga, Worthington, Reiland, Beauchaine, & Goldgar, 1985; Jerger & Mauldin, 1978; Prieve et al., 1993).

Most OAE data for neonates are available for TEOAEs (Brass & Kemp, 1994a, 1994b; Brass, Watkins, & Kemp, 1994; Kok et al., 1993; Maxon et al., 1995; Uziel & Piron, 1991; White et al., 1994), although data for neonate DPOAEs are becoming available (Bergman et al., 1995; Bonfils, Avan, Martine, Trotoux, & Narcy, 1992; Brown, Sheppard, & Russell, 1994; Lafreniere, Smurzynski, Jung, Leonard, & Kim, 1993; Spektor, Leonard, Kim, Jung, & Smurzynski, 1991). Reports suggest that otoacoustic emissions (OAE) may not adequately separate normal-hearing from impaired ears for frequencies below approximately 1000 Hz (Gorga et al., 1993b; 1994; Kim, Paparello, Jung, Smurzynski, & Sun, 1996; Prieve et al., 1993).

Specific characteristics (sensitivity, specificity, and predictive values) of test performance for ABR and OAE have not been fully defined in either universal or selective infant hearing screening applications (Joint Committee on Infant Hearing, 1994). For ABR, data suggest that test performance depends on the criteria that are chosen to define both hearing impairment and ABR outcome (Hyde et al, 1990). In addition, characteristics of the population to be screened (high risk vs. low risk) and the time of screening will affect test performance. For example, audiologists who design a screening program for healthy newborns who are to be discharged within 24 hours of birth should recognize that OAE test performance will be affected by the age at test. Kok et al., (1993) report that specificity of OAEs is lowest when conducted during the first 48 hours of life. In addition, external and middle ear status affect the OAE (Chang, Vohr, Norton, & Lekas, 1993; Osterhammel, Nielsen, & Rasmussen, 1993; Owens, McCoy, Lonsbury-Martin, & Martin, 1993; Trine, Hirsch, & Margolis, 1993; Vohr et al., 1996).

Follow-Up Procedures

Investigators have recommended a variety of follow-up protocols for infants referred from ABR or OAE screening. Recommendations include: (a) ABR screen followed immediately by threshold ABR for those referred from screening (Galambos et al., 1994; Stein et al., 1983); (b) OAE screen followed by ABR screen for those referred from screening (Kennedy et al., 1991; Stevens et al., 1989; and (c) OAE screen followed by OAE rescreen in 4 to 6 weeks for those referred from initial screening (Maxon et al., 1995). Factors that influence selection of a follow-up protocol include access to babies, cost, equipment, and personnel resources. Regardless of the selected protocol, follow-up procedures should ensure prompt completion of the diagnostic process and timely initiation of habilitative procedures.

Program Evaluation

The consequence of both false-negative and false-positive test results should be considered in the development of a newborn/very young infant hearing screening program. False-negative screening results may delay diagnosis of hearing impairment. [Reports from cystic fibrosis and mammography screening programs indicate that negative screening results significantly delay diagnosis and treatment (Henry, Boulton, & Roddick, 1990; Joensuu et al., 1994)]. Less emphasis has been placed on the impact of false-positive results on families. Although no research has been conducted to examine the impact of neonatal hearing screening results on families, reports from neonatal screening programs for phenylketonuria (PKU), hypothyroidism, cystic fibrosis, and metabolic disorders have described several adverse psychological and behavioral effects of false-positive results. These include parental responses of shock, sleep disturbances, maternal crying, and infant feeding problems, some of which remain even after subsequent testing results in negative findings (Bodegard, Fyro, & Larsson, 1982; Fyro & Bodegard, 1987; Levy, 1974; McBean, 1971; Sorenson, Levy, Mangione, & Sepe, 1984; Tluczek et al., 1992).

References

American Speech-Language-Hearing Association. (1981, March). Employment and utilization of supportive personnel in audiology and speech-language pathology. *Asha, 23,* 165–169.

American Speech-Language-Hearing Association. (1996, Spring). Scope of practice in audiology. *Asha, 38* (Suppl.16), 12–15.

Ballachanda, B. B., Roeser, R. J., & Kemp, R. J. (1996). Control and prevention of disease transmission in audiology practice. *American Journal of Audiology, 5* (1), 74–82.

Bergman, B. M., Gorga, M. P., Neely, S. T., Kaminski, J. K., Beauchaine, K. L., & Peters, J. (1995). Preliminary descriptions of transient-evoked and distortion-product otoacoustic emissions from graduates of an intensive care nursery. *Journal of American Academy of Audiology, 6,* 150–162.

Bess, F. H., Klee, T., & Culbertson, J. L. (1986). Identification, assessment, and management of children with unilateral sensorineural hearing loss. *Ear and Hearing, 7,* 43–51.

Bess, F. H., & Tharpe, A. M. (1986). Case history data on unilaterally hearing-impaired children. *Ear and Hearing, 7,* 14–19.

Bodegard, G., Fyro, K., & Larsson, A. (1982). Psychological reactions in 102 families with a newborn who has a falsely positive screening test for congenital hypothyroidism. *Acta Paediatrica Scandinavia,* (Suppl. 304), 1–21.

Bonfils, P., Avan, P., Martine, M., Trotoux, J., & Narcy, P. (1992). Distortion-product otoacoustic emissions in neonate: normative data. *Acta Otolaryngologica (Stockholm), 112,* 739–744.

Brass, D., & Kemp, D. T. (1994a). The objective assessment of transient evoked otoacoustic emissions in neonates. *Ear and Hearing, 15,* 371–377.

Brass, D., & Kemp, D. T. (1994b). Quantitative methods for the detection of otoacoustic emissions. *Ear and Hearing, 15,* 378–389.

Brass, D., Watkins, P., & Kemp, D. T. (1994). Assessment of an implementation of a narrow band neonatal otoacoustic emission screening method. *Ear and Hearing, 15,* 467–475.

Brown, A. M., Sheppard, S. L., & Russell, P. T. (1994). Acoustic distortion products (ADP) from the ears of term infants and young adults using low stimulus levels. *British Journal of Audiology, 28,* 273–280.

Chang, K. W., Vohr, B. R., Norton, S. J., & Lekas, M. D. (1993). External and middle ear status related to evoked otoacoustic emission in neonates. *Archives of Otolaryngology—Head and Neck Surgery, 119,* 276–282.

Coats, A. C., & Martin, J. L. (1977). Human auditory nerve action potentials and brainstem evoked responses: Effects of audiogram shape and lesion location. *Archives of Otolaryngology, 103,* 605–622.

Culbertson, J., & Gilbert, L. (1986). Children with unilateral sensorineural hearing loss: Cognitive, academic, and social development. *Ear and Hearing, 7,* 38–42.

Davis, A., Wood, S., Healy, R., Webb, H., & Rowe, S. (1995). Risk factors for hearing disorders: Epidemologic evidence of change over time in the UK. *Journal of American Academy of Audiology, 6,* 365–370.

Downs, M. P. (1967). Testing hearing in infancy and early childhood. In F. E. McConnell & P. H. Ward (Eds)., *Deafness in Childhood* (pp. 25–33). Nashville, TN: Vanderbilt University Press.

Durieux-Smith, A., Picton, T. W., Bernard, P., MacMurray, B., & Goodman, J. T. (1991). Prognostic validity of brainstem electric response audiometry in infants of a neonatal intensive care unit. *Audiology, 30,* 249–265.

Durieux-Smith, A., Picton, T., Edwards, C., Goodman, J., & MacMurray, B. (1985). The Crib-O-Gram in the NICU: An evaluation based on brainstem electric response audiometry. *Ear and Hearing, 6,* 20–24.

Fyro, K., & Bodegard, G. (1987). Four-year follow-up of psychological reactions to false-positive screening tests for congenital hypothyroidism. *Acta Paediatrica Scandinavia, 76,* 107–114.

Galambos, R., & Hecox, K. E. (1978). Clinical applications of the auditory brainstem response. *Otolaryngology Clinics of North America, 11,* 709–728.

Galambos, R., Wilson, M. J., & Silva, P. D. (1994). Identifying hearing loss in the intensive care nursery: A 20-year summary. *Journal of the American Academy of Audiology, 5,* 151–162.

Gaskill, S. A., & Brown, A. M. (1990). The behavior of the acoustic distortion product, 2f1–f2, from the human ear and its relation to auditory sensitivity. *Journal of the Acoustical Society of America, 88,* 821–839.

Gorga, M., Neely, S. T., Bergman, B., Beauchaine, K. L., Kaminski, J. R., Peters, J., & Jesteadt, W. (1993a). Otoacoustic emissions from normal-hearing and hearing impaired subjects: Distortion product responses. *Journal of the Acoustical Society of America, 93,* 2050–2060.

Gorga, M. P., Neely, S. T., Bergman, B., Beauchaine, K. L., Kaminski, J. R., Peters, J., Schulte, L., & Jesteadt, W. (1993b). A comparison of transient-evoked and distortion product otoacoustic emissions in normal-hearing and hearing impaired subjects. *Journal of the Acoustical Society of America, 94,* 2639–2648.

Gorga, M. P., Neely, S. T., Bergman, B., Beauchaine, K. L., Kaminski, J. R., & Liu, Z. (1994). Toward understanding the limits of distortion product otoacoustic emission measurements. *Journal of the Acoustical Society of America, 96* (3), 1494–1500.

Gorga, M., Worthington, D., Reiland, J., Beauchaine, K., & Goldgar, D. (1985). Some comparisons between auditory brainstem response thresholds, latencies, and the pure-tone audiogram. *Ear and Hearing, 5,* 247–253.

Hall, J. W. III. (1992). *Handbook of auditory evoked responses.* Boston: Allyn & Bacon.

Hall, J. W. III, Brown, D. P., & Mackay-Hargadine, J. (1985). Pediatric applications of serial auditory brainstem and middle latency measurements. *International Journal of Pediatric Otorhinolaryngology, 9,* 201–218.

Harris, F. P., Lonsbury-Martin, B. L., Stagner, B. B., Coats, A. C., & Martin, G. K. (1989). Acoustic distortion products in humans: Systematic changes in amplitude as a function of f2/f1 ratio. *Journal of the Acoustical Society of America, 85,* 220–229.

Henry, R. L., Boulton, T. J., & Roddick, L. G. (1990). False-negative results on newborn screening for cystic fibrosis. *Journal of Pediatrics and Child Health, 26,* 150–151.

Hosford-Dunn, H., Johnson, S., Simmons, F. B., Malachowski, N., & Low, K. (1987). Infant hearing screening: Program implementation and validation. *Ear and Hearing, 8,* 12–20.

Hyde, M., Riko, K., & Malizia, K. (1990). Audiometric accuracy of the click ABR in infants at risk for hearing loss. *Journal of the American Academy of Audiology, 1,* 59–66.

Jacobson, J. T., & Hall, J. W. III. (1994). Applications in newborn and infant auditory brainstem responses. In J. T. Jacobson (Ed.), *Principles and applications in auditory evoked potentials* (pp. 313–344). Boston: Allyn & Bacon.

Jacobson, J. T., Jacobson, C. A., & Spahr, R. C. (1990). Automated and conventional ABR screening techniques in high-risk infants. *Journal of the American Academy of Audiology, 1* (4), 187–195.

Jerger, J., & Mauldin, L. (1978). Prediction of sensorineural hearing level from the brainstem evoked response. *Archives of Otolaryngology, 104,* 656–661.

Joensuu, H., Asola, R., Holli, K., Kumpulainen, E., Nikkanen, V., & Parvinen, L. M. (1994). Delayed diagnosis and large size of breast cancer after a false-negative mammogram. *European Journal of Cancer, 30A,* 1299–1302.

Joint Committee on Infant Hearing. (1994, December). Position statement. *Asha, 36,* 38–41.

Katabamna, B., Bennett, S. L., Dokler, P. A., & Metz, D. A. (1995). Effects of electrode montage on infant auditory brainstem response. *Scandinavian Audiology, 24,* 133–136.

Kemp, D. T., & Ryan, S. (1993). The use of transient evoked otoacoustic emissions in neonatal hearing screening programs. *Seminars in Hearing, 14,* 30–45.

Kemp, D. T., Ryan, S., & Bray, P. (1990). A guide to the effective use of otoacoustic emissions. *Ear and Hearing, 11,* 93–105.

Kennedy, C. R., Kimm, L., Dees, D. C., Evans, P. I., Hunter, M., Lenton, S., & Thornton, R. D. (1991). Otoacoustic emissions and auditory brainstem responses in the newborn. *Archives of Disease in Childhood, 66,* 1124–1129.

Kim, D. O., Paparello, J., Jung, M. D., Smurzynski, J., & Sun, X. (1996). Distortion product otoacoustic emission test of sensorineural hearing loss: Performance regarding sensitivity, specificity and receiver operating characteristics. *Acta Otolaryngologica (Stockholm), 116,* 3–11.

Klee, T., & Davis-Dansky, E. (1986). A comparison of unilaterally hearing-impaired children and normal-hearing children on a battery of standardized language tests. *Ear and Hearing, 7,* 27–37.

Kok, M. R., van Zanten, G. A., Brocaar, M. P., & Wallenburg, H. C. S. (1993). Click-evoked otoacoustic emissions in 1036 ears of healthy newborns. *Audiology, 32,* 213–224.

Lafreniere, D., Smurzynski, J., Jung, M., Leonard, F., & Kim, D. O. (1993). Otoacoustic emissions in full-term newborns at risk for hearing loss. *Laryngoscope, 103,* 1334–1341.

Levy, H. L. (1974). Neonatal screening for inborn errors of metabolism. *Clinical Endocrinology and Metabolism, 3,* 153–166.

Mauk, G. W., White, K. R., Mortensen, L. B., & Behrens, T. R. (1991). The effectiveness of screening programs based on high-risk characteristics in early identification of hearing impairment. *Ear and Hearing, 12,* 312–319.

Maxon, A. B., White, K. R., Behrens, T. R., & Vohr, B. R. (1995). Referral rates and cost efficiency in a universal hearing screening program using transient evoked otoacoustic emissions. *Journal of American Academy of Audiology, 6,* 271–277.

McBean, M. S. (1971). The problems of parents of children with phenylketonuria. In J. Bickel, F. P. Hudson, & I. Woolf (Eds.), *Phenylketonuria and some other inborn errors of amino acid metabolism.* Stuttgart: Garig Thieme Verlag.

McCall, S., & Ferraro, J. A. (1991). Pediatric ABR screening: Pass-fail rates in awake versus asleep neonates. *Journal of the American Academy of Audiology, 2,* 18–23.

Mitchell, S. (1984). Noise pollution in the neonatal intensive care nursery. *Seminars in Hearing, 5* (1), 17–24.

National Institutes of Health. (1993). *Early identification of hearing impairment in infants and young children: Consensus Development Conference on Early Identification of Hearing Loss in Infants and Young Children* (Vol. 11). Bethesda, MD: NIH.

Osterhammel, P. A., Nielsen, L. H., & Rasmussen, A. N. (1993). Distortion product otoacoustic emissions: The influence of the middle ear transmission. *Scandinavian Audiology, 22,* 111–116.

Owens, J. J., McCoy, M. J., Lonsbury-Martin, B. L., & Martin, G. (1993). Otoacoustic emissions in children with normal ears, middle ear dysfunction, and ventilating tubes. *American Journal of Otology, 14* (1), 34–40.

Oyler, R. F., Oyler, A. L., & Matkin, N. D. (1987). Warning: A unilateral hearing loss may be detrimental to a child's academic career. *Hearing Journal, 40* (9), 18–22.

Oyler, R. F., Oyler, A. L., & Matkin, N. D. (1988). Unilateral hearing loss: Demographics and educational impact. *Language, Speech, and Hearing Services in Schools, 19,* 201–210.

Prieve, B. A., Gorga, M. P., Schmidt, A., Neely, S., Peters, J., Schultes, L., & Jesteadt, W. (1993). Analysis of transient-evoked otoacoustic emissions in normal-hearing and hearing-impaired ears. *Journal of the Acoustical Society of America, 93,* 3308–3319.

Sininger, Y. S. (1993). Auditory brainstem response for objective measures of hearing. *Ear and Hearing, 14* (1), 23–30.

Sininger, Y., Cone-Wesson, B., & Ma, E. (1994). Comparison of vertex-mastoid and vertical recording channels for ABR in human neonates. In G. R. Popelka (Ed.), *Abstracts of the Seventeenth Annual Midwinter Research Meeting of the Association for Research in Otolaryngology, 17,* 61.

Sininger, Y. S. (1995). Filtering and spectral characteristics of averaged auditory brainstem response and background noise in infants. *Journal of the Acoustical Society of America, 98,* 2048–2055.

Sorenson, J. R., Levy, H. L., Mangione, T. W., & Sepe, S. J. (1984). Parental response to repeat testing of infants with "false-positive" results in a newborn screening program. *Pediatrics, 73,* 183–187.

Spektor, Z., Leonard, G., Kim, D. O., Jung, M. D., & Smurzynski, J. (1991). Otoacoustic emissions in normal and hearing-impaired children and normal adults. *Laryngoscope, 101,* 965–976.

Stein, L., Ozdamar, O., Kraus, N., & Paton, J. (1983). Follow-up of infants screened by auditory brainstem response in the neonatal intensive care unit. *Journal of Pediatrics, 103,* 447–453.

Stevens, J. C., Webb, H. D., Hutchinson, J., Connell, J., Smith, M. F., & Buffin, J. T. (1989) Click evoked otoacoustic emissions compared to brainstem electric responses. *Archives of Disease in Childhood, 64,* 1105–1111.

Stover, L., Gorga, M. P., Neely, S. T., & Montoya, D. (1996). Toward optimizing the clinical utility of distortion product otoacoustic emission measurements. *Journal of the Acoustical Society of America, 100,* 956–967.

Stuart, A., & Yang, E. Y. (1994). Effect of high-pass filtering on the neonatal auditory brainstem response to ABR- and bone-conducted clicks. *Journal of Speech and Hearing Research, 37,* 475–479.

Tluczek, A., Micshler, E. H., Farrell, P. M., Fost, N., Peterson, N. M., & Carey, P. (1992). Parents' knowledge of neonatal screening and response to false-positive cystic fibrosis testing. *Developmental and Behavioral Pediatrics, 13,* 181–186.

Trine, M. B., Hirsch, J. E., & Margolis, R. H. (1993). Effect of middle ear pressure on transient evoked otoacoustic emissions. *Ear and Hearing, 14,* 401–407.

United States Department of Health and Human Services, Public Health Service, (1990). *Healthy People 2000: National health promotion and disease prevention objectives.* Washington, DC: US Government Printing Office.

U.S. Department of Labor, Occupational Safety and Health Administration. (1991, December 6). Occupational exposure to bloodborne pathogens: Final role. Washington, DC: *Federal Register.*

Uziel, A., & Piron, J. P. (1991). Evoked otoacoustic emissions from normal newborns and babies admitted to an intensive care baby unit. *Acta Otolaryngologica (Stockholm), 482,* 85–91.

Vohr, B. R., White, K. R., & Maxon, A. B. (1996). Effects of exam procedures on transient evoked otoacoustic emissions (TEOAEs) in neonates. *Journal of American Academy of Audiology, 7,* 77–82.

Vohr, B. R., White, K. R., Maxon, A. B., & Johnson, M. J. (1993). Factors affecting the interpretation of transient evoked otoacoustic emission results in neonatal hearing screening. *Seminars in Hearing, 14,* 57–72.

White, K. R., Vohr, B. R., & Behrens, T. R. (1993). Universal newborn hearing screening using transient evoked otoacoustic emissions: Results of the Rhode Island hearing assessment project. In T. R. Behrens & K. R.White (Eds.), The Rhode Island Hearing Assessment Project: Implications for universal newborn hearing screening. *Seminars in Hearing, 14,* 18–29.

White, K. R., Vohr, B. R., Maxon, A. B., Behrens, T. R., McPherson, M. G., & Mauk, G. W. (1994). Screening all newborns for hearing loss using transient evoked otoacoustic emissions. *International Journal of Pediatric Otorhinolaryngology, 29,* 203–217.

3. Guidelines for Screening for Hearing Impairment — Infants and Toddlers, 7 Months Through 2 Years

Specific guidelines for hearing screening of 7-month-old through 2-year-old children have not previously existed; however, assessment guidelines do exist (ASHA, 1991). Although this is a potentially difficult group to screen for hearing impairment, the Panel concluded that for this age group, the development of screening guidelines to be used only by audiologists was appropriate and necessary.

Infants and children who have not been screened in the first 6 months of life (Joint Committee on Infant Hearing, 1994) warrant hearing screening with the goal of detecting peripheral hearing impairment that may compromise cognitive development, communication, health, or future academic performance. Early detection of hearing impairment and intervention is possible. Screening procedures to detect hearing impairment that exceeds 20 to 30 dB HL are available and are applicable to this age group. Again, the Panel recommends using a pass-refer format to identify those children who require rescreening or complete audiologic evaluation. Optimally, those children who are referred from screening should have their hearing status confirmed within 1 month and no later than 3 months from the initial screening.

Developmental delays or extreme prematurity may limit application of screening methods that rely on behavioral responses. For those children unable to participate in behavioral procedures, screening methods used for the neonate through 6-month age group may be more appropriate (see previous set of guidelines).

The following outline contains the Panel's recommended guidelines for the development, supervision, and delivery of screening programs for hearing impairment in infants and toddlers (7 months through 2 years of age). The Panel provides a discussion of issues related to the rationale and assumptions underlying these recommendations. The Panel intends that this discussion section be fully considered prior to the implementation of the recommendations.

I. Personnel

Limit screening practitioners to audiologists with Certificate of Clinical Competence (CCC) from the American Speech-Language-Hearing Association (ASHA, 1996) and state licensure where applicable.

II. Expected Outcomes

Identification of infants and toddlers at risk for hearing impairment that may affect education, health, development, or communication.

III. Clinical Indications

A. Screen infants and toddlers as needed, requested, or mandated.

B. Screen infants and toddlers who have not previously received and passed hearing screening, or if they have indicators associated with congenital or acquired sensorineural and/or conductive hearing impairment (Joint Committee on Infant Hearing, 1994). Such indicators include:

1. parent/care provider and/or health care provider expresses concerns regarding hearing, speech, language, and/or developmental delay based on observation and/or standardized developmental screening (e.g., Early Language Milestone Scale, Coplan, 1987; Denver Developmental Screening Test-Revised [Denver II], Frankenburg, Dodds, Archer, Bresnick, & Shapiro, 1990);

2. craniofacial anomalies, including those with morphological abnormalities of the pinna and ear canal;

3. birth weight less than 1500 grams (3.3 lbs);

4. hyperbilirubinemia at a serum level requiring exchange transfusion;

5. ototoxic medications, including but not limited to chemotherapeutic agents or aminoglycosides, used in multiple courses or in combination with loop diuretics;

6. bacterial meningitis and other infections associated with sensorineural hearing loss;

7. Apgar scores of 0–4 at 1 minute or 0–6 at 5 minutes;

8. mechanical ventilation lasting 5 days or longer;

9. stigmata or other findings associated with a syndrome known to include sensorineural and/or conductive hearing loss;

10. head trauma associated with loss of consciousness or skull fracture;

11. family history of hereditary childhood sensorineural hearing loss;

12. in utero infection, such as cytomegalovirus, rubella, syphilis, herpes, and toxoplasmosis;

13. recurrent or persistent otitis media with effusion for at least 3 months;

14. neurofibromatosis type II or neurodegenerative disorders; and

15. anatomic disorders that affect eustachian tube function.

C. Some children may pass an initial hearing screening, but be at risk for fluctuating, delayed-onset, or progressive sensorineural and/or conductive hearing impairment. Those children's hearing should be monitored at least every 6 months until 3 years of age, and at regular intervals thereafter dependent on the risk factor (Joint Committee on Infant Hearing, 1994).

IV. Clinical Process

A. These guidelines recommend obtaining informed parental/legal guardian permission; however, extant state statutes or regulations, or institutional policies, supersede this recommendation.

B. Conduct screening in a manner congruent with infection control and universal precautions (Ballachanda, Roeser, & Kemp, 1996; U.S. Department of Labor, Occupational Safety and Health Administration, 1991).

C. For those children who can be conditioned for visual reinforcement audiometry (VRA), screen using earphones (conventional or insert), with 1000, 2000, and 4000 Hz tones at 30 dB HL (See discussion).

D. For those children who can be conditioned for play audiometry (CPA), screen using earphones (conventional or insert), with 1000, 2000, and 4000 Hz tones at 20 dB HL.

All hearing screening programs should include an educational component designed to provide parents with information, in lay language, on the process of hearing screening, the likelihood of their child having a hearing impairment, and follow-up procedures.

V. Pass/Refer Criteria

A. Pass if clinically reliable responses at criterion dB level at each frequency are present in each ear.

B. Refer if no response or no reliable response at criterion dB level at any frequency in either ear.

VI. Acceptable Modifications/Alternative Procedures

A. Screening in a calibrated sound field for those who do not accept earphone placement is acceptable; however, soundfield screening does not yield ear-specific information, and unilateral hearing loss may be missed.

B. EOAE or ABR may be employed to screen for hearing impairment. (See procedures described in the "Guidelines for Screening for Hearing Impairment—Newborns and Infants").

VII. Inappropriate Procedures

The following are not recommended:

A. noncalibrated signals, such as rattles, music boxes, noisemakers.

B. nonconditioned behavioral procedures, such as behavioral observation audiometry (BOA).

C. signals that lack frequency specificity, such as music, broadband noise.

D. speech stimuli in lieu of frequency-specific stimuli.

VIII. Follow-Up Procedures

A. A child who does not pass the screening should be rescreened or referred for audiologic evaluation dependent on the level of concern and professional judgment.

B. Confirmation of hearing status should be obtained within 1 month but no later than 3 months after the initial screening.

C. If possible, document follow-up results and personnel conducting follow-up.

XI. Setting/Equipment Specifications

A. Conduct screening in an environment, with minimal visual and auditory distractions, where ambient noise levels are sufficiently low to permit accurate measurements (ANSI, 1991).

B. Meet ANSI-S3.6 (ANSI, 1996) for all electroacoustic equipment.

C. Meet manufacturers' specification for calibration and regulatory agency specification for all equipment for electrical safety.

D. Conduct sound field testing in a sound-treated booth.

E. Calibrate audiometric equipment to ANSI S3.6 - 1996 specifications regularly, at least once every year, following the initial determination that the audiometer meets specifications. All the ANSI specifications, not just the sound pressure level, should be met.

F. Perform a daily listening check to rule out distortion, crosstalk, and intermittency, and to determine that no defects exist in major components.

X. Documentation

A. Record identifying information, screening results, and recommended follow-up procedures.

B. Request results from referral and follow-up.

Discussion

Personnel

Audiologists are the only professionals who have the knowledge, skill, and expertise to screen for hearing impairment in this age group.

Clinical Process

Two screening methods are suggested as the most appropriate tools for children who are functioning at 7 months to 3 years developmental age: visual reinforcement audiometry (VRA) and conditioned play audiometry (CPA). These two methods are both behavioral techniques that have proven track records with this age group. For children from approximately 6 months through 2 years of age, VRA is the recognized method of choice (ASHA, 1991; Primus & Thompson, 1985; Thompson & Folsom, 1984, 1985; Wilson & Moore, 1978). As children mature beyond their second birthday, CPA may be attempted (Nozza, 1995; Talbott, 1987; Thompson, Thompson, & Vethivelu, 1989).

Prior to initiating screening, the infant/child should be under stimulus control. A minimum of two conditioning trials at presumed suprathreshold levels should be completed before initiating screening. Screening stimuli are presented a minimum of two times at each frequency.

For VRA, the suggested stimulus level is 30 dB HL, and for CPA, it is 20 dB HL. The rationale for these different levels is two-fold. First, children who can perform CPA are more likely to give higher at-tention to the task than the children who require VRA. Second, detection thresholds in young children are elevated (Nozza, 1995; Nozza & Wilson, 1984). It should be noted, however, that the use of a higher level for the VRA group compromises the detection of hearing impairment at less than the criterion level.

Acceptable Modifications/Alternative Procedures

When a child refuses earphone placement or earphone placement is otherwise precluded, stimuli are presented in the sound field. When this occurs, ear-specific information is lacking, and unilateral hearing impairment will be missed. Parents should be advised that unilateral hearing impairment is not ruled out for these children.

Evoked otoacoustic emissions (OAE) are suggested as an alternative procedure when behavioral methods are ineffective. It should be recognized that external and middle ear status affect the EOAE (Chang, Vohr, Norton, & Lekas, 1993; Osterhammel, Nielsen, & Rasmussen, 1993; Owens, McCoy, Lonsbury-Martin, & Martin, 1993; Trine, Hirsch, & Margolis, 1993). Data on applying EOAE screening to this age group is lacking; however, much OAE data are available for neonates, young infants, older children, and adults that may be cautiously generalized to children in this age range (Bergman et al., 1995; Engdahl, Arnesen, & Mair, 1994; Glattke, Pafitis, Cummiskey, & Herer, 1995; Prieve et al., 1993; Smurzynski, Leonard, Kim, Lafreniere, & Jung, 1990; Spektor, Leonard, Kim, Jung, & Smurzynski, 1991). Reports suggest that evoked otoacoustic emissions (EOAE) may not adequately separate normal-hearing from impaired ears for frequencies below approximately 1000 Hz (Gorga et al., 1993, 1994; Kim, Paparello, Jung, Smurzynski, & Sun, 1996; Prieve et al., 1993).

References

American National Standards Institute. (1991). *Maximum permissible ambient noise levels for audiometric test rooms* (ANSI S3.1-1991). New York: Acoustical Society of America.

American National Standards Institute. (1996). *Specifications for audiometers* (ANSI S3.6-1996). New York: Acoustical Society of America.

American Speech-Language-Hearing Association. (1991, March). The guidelines for the audiologic assessment of children from birth through 36 months of age. *Asha, 33* (Suppl. 5), 37–43.

American Speech-Language-Hearing Association. (1996, Spring). Scope of practice in audiology. *Asha, 38* (Suppl. 16), 12–15.

Ballachanda, B. B., Roeser, R. J., & Kemp, R. J. (1996). Control and prevention of disease transmission in audiology practice. *American Journal of Audiology, 5* (1), 74–82.

Bergman, B. M., Gorga, M. P., Neely, S. T., Kaminski, J. K., Beauchaine, K. L., & Peters, J. (1995). Preliminary descriptions of transient-evoked and distortion-product otoacoustic emissions from graduates of an intensive care nursery. *Journal of American Academy of Audiology, 6,* 150–162.

Chang, K. W., Vohr, B. R., Norton, S. J., & Lekas, M. D. (1993). External and middle ear status related to evoked otoacoustic emission in neonates. *Archives of Otolaryngology—Head and Neck Surgery, 119,* 276–282.

Coplan, J. (1987). *Early Language Milestone Scale.* Austin, TX: Pro-ED.

Engdahl, B., Arnesen, A. R., & Mair, I. W. S. (1994). Otoacoustic emissions in the first year of life. *Scandinavian Audiology, 23,* 195–200.

Frankenburg, W. K., Dodds, J., Archer, P., Bresnick, B., & Shapiro, H. (1990). The Denver II: Revision and restandardization of the DDST. *American Journal of Diseases in Childhood, 144,* 446.

Glattke, T. J., Pafitis, I. A., Cummiskey, C., & Herer, G. R. (1995). Identification of hearing loss in children and young adults using measures of transient otoacoustic emission reproducibility. *American Journal of Audiology, 4* (3), 71–85.

Gorga, M. P., Neely, S. T., Bergman, B., Beauchaine, K. L., Kaminski, J. R., Peters, J., & Jesteadt, W. (1993). Otoacoustic emissions from normal-hearing and hearing impaired subjects: Distortion product responses. *Journal of the Acoustical Society of America, 93,* 2050–2060.

Gorga, M. P., Neely, S. T., Bergman, B., Beauchaine, K. L., Kaminski, J. R., & Liu, Z. (1994). Toward understanding the limits of distortion product otoacoustic emission measurements. *Journal of the Acoustical Society of America, 96* (3), 1494–1500.

Joint Committee on Infant Hearing. (1994, December). Position statement. *Asha, 36,* 38–41.

Kim, D. O., Paparello, J., Jung, M. D., Smurzynski, J., & Sun, X. (1996). Distortion product otoacoustic emission test of sensorineural hearing loss: Performance regarding sensitivity, specificity and receiver operating characteristics. *Acta Otolaryngologica (Stockholm), 116,* 3–11.

Nozza, R. J. (1995). Estimating the contribution of nonsensory factors to infant-adult differences in behavioral thresholds. *Hearing Research, 91,* 72–78.

Nozza, R. J., & Wilson, W. R. (1984). Masked and unmasked pure-tone thresholds of infants and adults: Development of auditory frequency selectivity and sensitivity. *Journal of Speech and Hearing Research, 27,* 613–622.

Osterhammel, P. A., Nielsen, L. H., & Rasmussen, A. N. (1993). Distortion product otoacoustic emissions: The influence of the middle ear transmission. *Scandinavian Audiology, 22,* 111–116.

Owens, J. J., McCoy, M. J., Lonsbury-Martin, B. L., & Martin, G. (1993). Otoacoustic emissions in children with normal ears, middle ear dysfunction, and ventilating tubes. *American Journal of Otology, 14* (1), 34–40.

Prieve, B. A., Gorga, M. P., Schmidt, A., Neely, S., Peters, J., Schultes, L., & Jesteadt, W. (1993). Analysis of transient-evoked otoacoustic emissions in normal-hearing and hearing-impaired ears. *Journal of the Acoustical Society of America, 93,* 3308–3319.

Primus, M. A., & Thompson, G. (1985). Response strength of young children in operant audiometry. *Journal of Speech and Hearing Research, 28,* 539–547.

Smurzynski, J., Leonard, G., Kim, D. O., Lafreniere, D. C., & Jung, M. D. (1990). Distortion product otoacoustic emissions in normal and impaired adult ears. *Archives of Otolaryngology—Head and Neck Surgery, 116,* 1309–1316.

Spektor, Z., Leonard, G., Kim, D. O., Jung, M. D., & Smurzynski, J. (1991). Otoacoustic emissions in normal and hearing-impaired children and normal adults. *Laryngoscope, 101,* 965–976.

Talbott, C. B. (1987). A longitudinal study comparing responses of hearing-impaired infants to pure tones using visual reinforcement and play audiometry. *Ear and Hearing, 8,* 175–179.

Thompson, G., & Folsom, R. C. (1984). A comparison of two conditioning procedures in the use of visual reinforcement audiometry (VRA). *Journal of Speech and Hearing Disorders, 49,* 241–245.

Thompson, G., & Folsom, R. C. (1985). Reinforced and nonreinforced head-turn responses of infants as a function of stimulus bandwidth. *Ear and Hearing, 6,* 125–129.

Thompson, M., Thompson, G., & Vethivelu, S. (1989). A comparison of audiometric test methods for 2-year-old children. *Journal of Speech and Hearing Disorders, 50,* 174–179.

Trine, M. B., Hirsch, J. E., & Margolis, R. H. (1993). The effect of middle ear pressure on transient evoked otoacoustic emissions. *Ear and Hearing, 14,* 401–407.

U.S. Department of Labor, Occupational Safety and Health Administration (1991, December 6). Occupational exposure to bloodborne pathogens: Final rule. Washington, DC: *Federal Register.*

Wilson, W. R., & Moore, J. M. (1978). *Pure-tone earphone thresholds of infants utilizing visual reinforcement audiometry (VRA).* Paper presented at the ASHA Convention, San Francisco.

4. Guidelines for Screening for Hearing Impairment— Preschool Children, 3 to 5 Years

Previous guidelines for screening for hearing impairment in the 3- to 5-year-old age group were included in guidelines for school age children (ASHA, 1985, 1990). The Panel decided to develop separate guidelines for this age group because the testing procedure used for this age, specifically conditioned play audiometry, requires more training, instruction, and caution on the part of the examiner than do traditional screening procedures used with older children.

The goal of screening for hearing impairment is to identify the preschool children most likely to have peripheral hearing impairment that may interfere with communication, development, health, or future academic performance. In addition, because the preponderance of hearing impairments identified in this age range are associated with middle ear disease, the Panel recommends that children in this age group concurrently be screened for hearing disorder (refer to pediatric guideline for screening for outer and middle ear disorders). The goal of screening for middle ear disorder in this age range is to identify preschool children at risk of developing hearing impairment and/or medical conditions that warrant attention.

Screening for hearing impairment is a pass-refer procedure to identify individuals who require further audiologic evaluation or other assessments. Hearing impairment is defined as unilateral or bilateral sensorineural and/or conductive hearing loss greater than 20 dB HL in the frequency region from 1000 through 4000 Hz.

Developmental delay or behavioral reticence may preclude the use of the play audiometry procedures suggested here, in which case the screening methods used for the infant-toddler group may be more appropriate. Refer to "Guidelines for Screening for Hearing Impairment—Infants and Toddlers, 7 Months Through 2 Years." Likewise, school-age procedures may be appropriate for the more mature preschoolers ("Guidelines for Screening for Hearing Impairment—School-Age Children, 5 Through 18 Years ").

The following outline contains the Panel's recommended guidelines for the development, supervision, and delivery of screening programs for hearing impairment in children 3 to 5 years of age. The Panel provides a discussion of issues related to the rationale and assumptions underlying the recommendations. The Panel intends that this discussion section be considered fully prior to the implementation of these recommendations.

I. Personnel

Screening practitioners should be limited to:

A. Audiologists holding a Certificate of Clinical Competence (CCC-A) from the American Speech-Language-Hearing Association (ASHA) and state licensure where applicable (ASHA, 1996a).

B. Speech-language pathologists holding a Certificate of Clinical Competence (CCC-SLP) from the American Speech-Language-Hearing Association (ASHA) and state licensure where applicable (ASHA, 1996b).

C. Support personnel under supervision of a certified audiologist (ASHA, 1981).

II. Expected Outcomes

Identification of preschool children at risk for hearing impairment that may affect communication and development.

III. Clinical Indications

A. Preschool children are screened as needed, requested, or mandated, or when they have conditions that place them at risk for hearing impairment.

B. Indicators associated with delayed-onset, progressive or acquired sensorineural and/or conductive hearing impairment include:

1. parent/care provider and/or health care provider concerns regarding hearing, speech, language, and/or developmental delay based on observation and/or standardized develop-

mental screening (e.g., Denver Developmental Screening Test—Revised [Denver II], Frankenburg, Dodds, Archer, Bresnick, & Shapiro, 1990);

2. family history of hereditary childhood hearing loss;

3. in utero infection, such as cytomegalovirus, rubella, syphilis, herpes, and toxoplasmosis;

4. craniofacial anomalies, including those with morphological abnormalities of the pinna and ear canal;

5. ototoxic medications, including but not limited to the aminoglycosides, used in multiple courses or in combination with loop diuretics;

6. bacterial meningitis and other infections associated with sensorineural hearing loss;

7. stigmata or other findings associated with a syndrome known to include sensorineural and/or conductive hearing loss;

8. head trauma associated with loss of consciousness or skull fracture;

9. neurofibromatosis type II or neurodegenerative disorders; and

10. recurrent or persistent otitis media with effusion for at least 3 months.

IV. Clinical Process

A. These guidelines recommend obtaining informed parental/legal guardian permission; however, extant state statutes or regulations, or institutional policies, supersede this recommendation.

B. Conduct screening in a manner congruent with appropriate infection control and universal precautions (Ballachanda, Roeser, & Kemp, 1996; U.S. Department of Labor, Occupational Safety and Health Administration, 1991).

C. Condition the child to the desired motor response prior to initiation of screening. Administer a minimum of two conditioning trials at a presumed suprathreshold level to assure that the child understands the task.

D. If child can reliably participate in conditioned play audiometry (CPA) or conventional audiometry, screen under earphones (conventional or insert earphones), using 1000, 2000, and 4000 Hz tones at 20 dB HL.

E. At least two presentations of each test stimulus may be required to assure reliability.

F. All hearing screening programs should include an educational component designed to provide parents with information, in lay language, on the process of hearing screening, the likelihood of their child having a hearing impairment, and follow-up procedures.

V. Pass/Refer Criteria

A. Pass if child's responses are judged to be clinically reliable at least 2 out of 3 times at the criterion decibel level at each frequency in each ear.

B. Refer if child does not respond at least 2 out of 3 times at the criterion decibel level at any frequency in either ear or if the child cannot be conditioned to the task.

VI. Acceptable Modifications/Alternative Procedures

A. Screening in the sound field for those who do not accept earphone placement is acceptable, however, this precludes identification of unilateral hearing impairments.

B. For those preschool children who cannot be conditioned for play audiometry, screen by visual reinforcement audiometry (VRA).

VII. Inappropriate Procedures

Signals that lack frequency specificity (e.g., speech, music, broad-band noise).

VIII. Follow-Up Procedures

A. If referral is attributable to failure to condition, screen using infant-toddler procedures (see "Guidelines for Screening For Hearing Impairments—Infants and Toddlers, 7 Months Through 2 Years") or recommend for audiologic assessment.

B. If referral is not attributable to failure to condition, recommend audiologic assessment.

C. Confirm hearing status of children referred within 1 month but no later than 3 months after the initial screening.

IX. Setting/Equipment Specifications

A. Conduct screening in a clinical or natural environment, with minimal visual and auditory distractions. Ambient noise levels must be sufficiently low to allow for accurate screening (American National Standards Institute, 1991).

B. Meet ANSI and manufacturer's specification for calibration (American National Standards Institute, 1996) and regulatory agency specification for electrical safety for all electroacoustic equipment.

C. Calibrate audiometers to ANSI S3.6-1996 specifications regularly, at least once every year, following the initial determination that the audiometer meets specifications. All the ANSI specifications, not just the sound pressure level, should be met.

D. Perform a daily listening check to rule out distortion, cross talk, and intermittency, and to determine that no defects exist in major components.

X. Documentation

A. Record identifying information, screening results, and recommended follow-up procedures.

B. Request results from referral and follow-up.

Discussion

Unlike the newborn and school age populations, where nearly all children are accessible in hospitals and schools, preschoolers are generally not available in large, organized groups that lend themselves to universal screening for hearing impairment. For this reason, an interdisciplinary, collaborative effort is particularly important for this age group. Physicians and other professionals who specialize in child development should be included in the planning and implementation of the hearing screening program to maximize the likelihood of prompt referral of children at risk of hearing impairment and care of children referred from screening.

Clinical Process

Conditioned Play Audiometry (CPA) is the most commonly employed behavioral audiometric procedure for preschool children (Lowell, Rushford, Hoversten, & Stoner, 1956; Mahoney, 1992; O'Neill, Oyer, & Hillis, 1961). It is a form of instrumental/operant conditioning in which the child is taught to wait and listen for a stimulus, then perform a motor task in response to the stimulus. The motor task is a play activity, which serves as reinforcement.

References

American National Standards Institute. (1991). *Maximum permissible ambient noise levels for audiometric test rooms* (ANSI S3.1-1991). New York: Acoustical Society of America.

American National Standards Institute. (1996). *Specifications for audiometers* (ANSI S3.6-1996). New York: Acoustical Society of America.

American Speech-Language-Hearing Association. (1981). Guidelines for the employment and utilization of supportive personnel. *Asha, 23* (3), 165–169.

American Speech-Language-Hearing Association. (1985, May). Guidelines for identification audiometry. *Asha, 27*, 49–52.

American Speech-Language-Hearing Association. (1990, April). Guidelines for screening for hearing impairment and middle-ear disorders. *Asha, 32* (Suppl. 2), 17–24.

American Speech-Language-Hearing Association. (1996a, Spring). Scope of practice in audiology. *Asha, 38* (Suppl. 16), 12–15.

American Speech-Language-Hearing Association. (1996b, Spring). Scope of practice in speech-language pathology. *Asha, 38* (Suppl. 16), 1–4

Ballachanda, B. B., Roeser, R. J., & Kemp, R. J. (1996). Control and prevention of disease transmission in audiology practice. *American Journal of Audiology, 5* (1), 74–82.

Fluharty, N. B. (1978). The design and standardization of a speech and language screening test for use with preschool children. *Journal of Speech and Hearing Disorders, 39*, 75–88.

Frankenburg, W. K., Dodds, J., Archer, P., Bresnick, B., & Shapiro, H. (1990). The Denver II: Revision and restandardization of the DDST. *American Journal of Diseases in Childhood, 144*, 446.

Lowell, E., Rushford, G., Hoversten, G., & Stoner, M. (1956). Evaluation of pure tone audiometry with preschool age children. *Journal of Speech and Hearing Disorders, 21*, 292–302.

Mahoney, T. (1992). Screening the preschool-age child. In F. H. Bess & J. W. Hall III (Eds.) *Screening children for auditory function* (pp. 273–294). Nashville: Bill Wilkerson Center Press.

O'Neill, J., Oyer, H. J., & Hillis, J. W. (1961). Audiometric procedures used with children. *Journal of Speech and Hearing Disorders, 26*, 61–66.

U.S. Department of Labor, Occupational Safety and Health Administration (1991, December 6). Occupational exposure to bloodborne pathogens: Final rule. Washington, DC: *Federal Register*.

5. Guidelines for Screening for Hearing Impairment— School-Age Children, 5 Through 18 Years

Screening for hearing impairment identifies school-age children most likely to have peripheral hearing impairment that may interfere with education, health, development, or communication. It is a pass/refer procedure used to identify those children who require further audiologic evaluation. For school-age children, hearing impairment is defined as unilateral or bilateral sensorineural and/or conductive hearing loss greater than 20 dB HL in the frequency region most important for speech recognition (approximately 500 to 4000 Hz).

The outline presented below contains the Panel's recommended guidelines for the development, supervision, and delivery of screening programs for hearing impairment in school-aged children. The Panel provides a discussion of important issues related to the rationale and assumptions underlying the recommendations. The Panel intends that this discussion section be considered fully prior to the implementation of its recommendations.

I. Personnel

Limit screening practitioners to:

A. Audiologists holding a Certificate of Clinical Competence (CCC-A) from the American Speech-Language-Hearing Association (ASHA) and state licensure where applicable (ASHA, 1996a).

B. Speech-language pathologists holding a Certificate of Clinical Competence (CCC-SLP) from the American Speech-Language-Hearing Association (ASHA) and state licensure where applicable (ASHA, 1996b).

C. Support personnel under supervision of a certified audiologist (ASHA, 1981).

II. Expected Outcome

Identification of school children at risk for hearing impairment that may affect adversely education, health, development, or communication.

III. Clinical Indications

A. Screen school-age children on initial entry to school, and annually in kindergarten through 3rd grade, and in 7th and 11th grades.

B. Screen school-age children as needed, requested, or mandated. Additionally, children should be screened upon entrance to special education, or grade repetition, or new entry to the school system without evidence of having passed a previous hearing screening, or absence during a previously scheduled screening.

C. The following risk factors suggest the need for a hearing screening in other years:

1. parent/care provider, health care provider, teacher, or other school personnel have concerns regarding hearing, speech, language, or learning abilities;

2. family history of late or delayed onset hereditary hearing loss;

3. recurrent or persistent otitis media with effusion for at least 3 months;

4. craniofacial anomalies, including those with morphological abnormalities of the pinna and ear canal;

5. stigmata or other findings associated with a syndrome known to include sensorineural and/or conductive hearing loss;

6. head trauma with loss of consciousness;

7. reported exposure to potentially damaging noise levels or ototoxic drugs.

D. School-age children who receive regular audiologic management need not participate in a screening program.

IV. Clinical Process

A. These guidelines recommend obtaining informed consent, or, in the case of children, informed parental/legal guardian permission; however, extant state statutes or regulations, or institutional policies, supersede this recommendation.

B. Conduct screening in a manner congruent with appropriate infection control and universal precautions (Ballachanda, Roeser, & Kemp, 1996; U.S. Department of Labor, OSHA, 1991).

C. Conditioned play audiometry (CPA) or conventional audiometry are the procedures of choice.

D. Conduct screening under earphones using 1000, 2000, and 4000 Hz tones at 20 dB HL (See "Setting/Equipment Specifications").

E. All hearing screening programs should include an educational component designed to provide parents with information, in lay language, on the process of hearing screening, the likelihood of their child having a hearing impairment, and follow-up procedures.

V. Pass/Refer Criteria

A. Pass if responses are judged to be clinically reliable at criterion dB level at each frequency in each ear.

B. If a child does not respond at criterion dB level at any frequency in either ear, reinstruct, reposition earphones, and rescreen within the same screening session in which the child fails.

C. Pass children who pass the rescreening.

D. Refer children who fail the rescreening or fail to condition to the screening task.

VI. Inappropriate Procedures

The following are not recommended:

A. speech stimuli in lieu of frequency-specific stimuli;

B. nonconventional instrumentation, such as hand-held devices;

C. noncalibrated signals (e.g., noisemakers, whisper);

D. group screening procedures; and

E. transient evoked otoacoustic emissions (TEOAE) or distortion product otoacoustic emissions (DPOAE) testing.

VII. Follow-Up Procedures

A. If referred for hearing impairment, recommend audiologic assessment. Confirm the hearing status of referred children optimally within 1 month but no later than 3 months after initial screening.

VIII. Setting/Equipment Specifications

A. Conduct screening in a sound-treated booth or a quiet environment, with minimal visual and auditory distractions.

B. For screening environments, ambient noise levels should not exceed 49.5 dB SPL at 1000 Hz, 54.5 dB SPL at 2000 Hz, and 62 dB SPL at 4000 Hz when measured using a sound level meter with octave-band filters centered on the screening frequencies. These levels are derived from consideration of ANSI (1991) standards for pure-tone threshold testing, and are adjusted for the 20 dB HL screening level.

C. Use audiometers that meet ANSI S3.6-1996 requirements for either limited range or narrow-range audiometers.

D. Calibrate to ANSI S3.6-1996 specifications regularly, at least once every year, following the initial determination that the audiometer meets specifications. All the ANSI specifications, not just the sound pressure level, should be met.

E. Perform a daily listening check to rule out distortion, crosstalk, and intermittency, and to determine that no defects exist in major components.

F. Use electroacoustic equipment that meets regulatory agency specification for electrical safety.

IX. Documentation

A. Document identifying information, screening results, and recommendations for rescreening, assessment, or referral.

B. Record information pertaining to follow-up, including personnel conducting follow-up.

C. Prior to initiating screening, arrange process for notifying parent/guardian of the screening result.

Discussion

Clinical Process

School-age children with even minimal hearing impairments are at risk for academic and communicative difficulties (Tharpe & Bess, 1991). Due to the critical importance of identifying school-age children with minimal hearing impairments, the panel recommends a minimal screening level of 20 dB HL.

In this guideline, the schedule of recommended screenings reflects a change from previous screening documents. The Panel based its recommended schedule on these factors: (a) the apparently increased potential for hearing loss among adolescents due to overexposure to high levels of noise, and (b) the critical importance of identifying older school-age children at risk for hearing impairment that may affect their future educational, vocational, or social opportunities in the adult world. (Montgomery & Fujikawa, 1992; Peppard & Peppard, 1992).

Intermediate hearing screening occurring after an initial screen at school entry has never been evaluated for their yield. It is strongly recommended that an examination on the incremental yield of each screening stage be the focus of future research endeavors (Haggard, 1992).

Inappropriate Procedures

Hand-held devices are not recommended in the school-age population based on the high false positive rate (Bess, Dodd Murphy, & Parker, submitted).

Information on transient evoked otoacoustic emissions (TEOAE) and distortion product otoacoustic emissions (DPOAE) as screening tools in the school-age population is limited. Current available data suggest that these are promising procedures for the future of screening for hearing disorder in this population (Nozza & Sabo, 1992; Nozza, Sabo, & Mandel, in press); however, they are not recommended for use at this time.

Follow-Up Procedures

Appropriate management and follow-up of children who do not pass the hearing screening is of utmost importance to the efficacy of the screening program. If a child is referred based on the results of his or her rescreening, a process for notifying the parent/guardian should be implemented that provides information, in lay language, regarding the meaning of the referral and the recommended follow-up procedures.

A major component of a screening program for school-aged children is educating the student and school personnel. The teacher of any student found to have a hearing impairment should receive appropriate instruction and consultation regarding the potential psychoeducational impact of hearing loss. Classroom teachers should be provided with management strategies to assist identified students during instructional times and extracurricular activities, such as preferential seating, speaking at a slower rate, study buddies, and speaking face-to-face (Edwards, 1996; Matkin & Sturgeon, 1992).

Another major educational responsibility of the audiologist is to provide information to students regarding the potential deleterious effects that overexposure to high levels of all types of sounds can have on hearing (i.e., loud music, industrial arts class, tar-

get practice, etc.). Such an educational program is extremely important in the prevention of permanent noise-induced hearing impairments.

References

American National Standards Institute. (1991). *Maximum permissible ambient noise levels for audiometric test rooms* (ANSI S3.1-1991). New York: Acoustical Society of America.

American National Standards Institute. (1996). *Specifications for audiometers* (ANSI S3.6-1996). New York: Acoustical Society of America.

American Speech-Language-Hearing Association. (1981, March). Guidelines for the employment and utilization of supportive personnel. *Asha, 23* (3), 165–169.

American Speech-Language-Hearing Association. (1996a, Spring). Scope of practice in audiology. *Asha, 38* (Suppl. 16), 12–15.

American Speech-Language-Hearing Association. (1996b, Spring). Scope of practice in speech-language pathology. *Asha, 38* (Suppl. 16), 1–4.

Ballachanda, B. B., Roeser, R. J., & Kemp, R. J. (1996). Control and prevention of disease transmission in audiology practice. *American Journal of Audiology, 5* (1), 74–82.

Bess, F. H., Dodd Murphy, J., & Parker, R. A. (submitted). Children with minimal sensorineural hearing: Prevalence, educational performance, and functional status.

Edwards, C. (1996). Auditory intervention for children with mild auditory deficits. In F. Bess, J. Gravel, & A. M. Tharpe (Eds.), *Amplification for children with auditory deficits*. Nashville, TN: Bill Wilkerson Center Press.

Haggard, M. (1992). Screening children's hearing. *British Journal of Audiology, 26,* 209–215.

Montgomery, J. K., & Fujikawa, S. (1992). Hearing thresholds of students in 2nd, 8th, and 12th grades. *Language, Speech, and Hearing Services in Schools, 23,* 61–63.

Matkin, N. D., & Sturgeon, J. (1992). Guidelines for the classroom teacher serving the hearing-impaired child. In F. Bess & J. W. Hall III (Eds.), *Screening children for auditory function*. Nashville, TN: Bill Wilkerson Center.

Nozza, R. J., & Sabo, D. L. (1992). Transient evoked OAE for screening school-age children. *Hearing Journal, 45* (11), 29–31.

Nozza, R. J., Sabo, D. L., & Mandel, E. M. (in press). A role for otoacoustic emissions in screening for hearing impairment and middle ear disorder in school age children. *Ear and Hearing.*

Peppard, A. R., & Peppard, S. B. (1992). Noise-induced hearing loss: A study of children at risk. *Hearing Journal, 45,* 33–35.

Tharpe, A. M. & Bess, F. H. (1991). Identification and management of children with minimal hearing loss. *International Journal of Pediatric Otorhinolaryngology, 21,* 41–50.

U.S. Department of Labor, Occupational Safety and Health Administration (1991, December 6). Occupational exposure to bloodborne pathogens: Final rule. Washington, DC: *Federal Register.*

6. Guidelines for Screening for Disability in Children—Birth Through 18 Years

Screening for hearing disability in children has two purposes. First, screening for hearing disability permits referral of those children who exhibit delays in the development of communication milestones. The disabilities generally screened for include speech/language development, academic, or behavior problems. Second, for children already identified as having hearing impairment, screening and subsequent assessment for disability should be viewed as part of overall audiological management.

The outline provided below contains the Panel's recommendations for the screening of hearing disability in children.

I. Personnel

Although specific tools may dictate the appropriate personnel to administer the screening, the range of currently available tools allow screening practitioners to include:

A. Audiologists with a Certificate of Clinical Competence (CCC-A) from the American Speech-Language-Hearing Association (ASHA) and state licensure where applicable (ASHA, 1996a).

B. Speech-language pathologists with a Certificate of Clinical Competence (CCC-SLP) from the American Speech-Language-Hearing Association (ASHA) and state licensure where applicable (ASHA, 1996b).

C. Physicians, nurses, educators, or other personnel.

II. Expected Outcomes

Identification of those children most likely to have hearing disabilities that interfere with their social, educational, vocational performance, and communication.

III. Clinical Indications

A. Screen infants, toddlers, and school-age children as needed, requested, mandated, or when they have conditions that place them at risk for hearing disability.

B. Screen all infants and young children at well-baby visits to physician offices and clinics and during audiological evaluations. For the birth to 60-month age range, the Committee on Practice and Ambulatory Medicine in consultation with the American Academy of Pediatrics (1995) has recommended postnatal well-baby visits at 1, 2, 4, 6, 9, 12, 15, 18, 24, 36, 48, and 60 months. At later well-child visits, child should be screened if parent/caregiver expresses concern.

IV. Clinical Process

A. These guidelines recommend obtaining informed consent, or, in the case of children, informed parental/legal guardian permission; however, extant state statutes or regulations, or institutional policies, supersede this recommendation.

B. The following are examples of instruments commonly used to screen for disability by age group:

• For the infant and toddler population: the Communication Screen (Striffler & Willis, 1981), the Early Language Milestone Scale (ELM) (Coplan, 1983), the Fluharty Preschool Speech and Language Screening Test (Fluharty, 1974), and the Physician's Developmental Quick Screen for Speech Disorders (Kulig & Bakler, 1973).

• For the preschool population: the Communication Screen (Striffler & Willis, 1981), the Compton Speech and Language Screening Evaluation (Compton, 1978), the Physician's Developmental Quick Screen for Speech Disorders (Kulig & Bakler, 1973), the Texas Preschool Screening Inventory (Haber & Norris, 1983), the Fluharty Preschool Speech and Language Screening Test (Fluharty, 1974), and the Preschool SIFTER (Anderson & Matkin, 1996).

• For the school-age population: the SIFTER (Anderson, 1989).

C. Children with known hearing impairment should receive evaluation for disability. It is appropriate, however, to screen for disability in specific settings (i.e., in the educational setting).

V. Pass/Refer Criteria

Criteria for referral depend on the specific tool used.

VI. Inappropriate Procedures

Do not use measures that do not offer published data regarding internal consistency/reliability, test-retest reliability, and pass/fail criteria. For a comprehensive review of preschool speech and language screening tools, see Sturner, Layton, Evans, Funk, and Machon (1994).

VII. Follow-Up Procedures

Positive findings should result in referral to audiologists, speech-language pathologists, early intervention specialists, local education agencies, or other professionals as appropriate.

VIII. Setting/Instrument Specifications

Use any quiet environment conducive to interview/screening.

IX. Documentation

A. Document identifying information, screening results, and recommendations for follow-up procedures.

B. If possible, document follow-up results and personnel conducting follow-up.

References

American Speech-Language-Hearing Association. (1996a, Spring). Scope of practice in audiology. *Asha, 38* (Suppl. 16), 12–15.

American Speech-Language-Hearing Association. (1996b, Spring). Scope of practice in speech-language pathology. *Asha, 38* (Suppl. 16), 1–4.

Anderson, K. L. (1989). *Screening Instrument for Targeting Educational Risk (SIFTER)*. Austin, TX: Pro-Ed.

Anderson, K. L., & Matkin, N. D. (1996). *Preschool SIFTER: Screening instrument for targeting educational risk in preschool children (age 3–kindergarten)*. Tampa, FL: Educational Audiology Association.

Capute, A. J., Palmer, F. B., Shapiro, B. K., et al. (1986). The clinical linguistic and auditory milestone scale of infancy (CLAMS): Prediction of cognition in infancy. *Developmental Medicine and Child Neurology, 28*, 762–771.

Committee on Practice and Ambulatory Medicine. (1995). Recommendations for preventive pediatric health care. *Pediatrics, 96*(2).

Compton, A. (1978). *Compton Speech and Language Screening Evaluation*. San Francisco: Carousel House.

Coplan, J. (1983). *ELM Scale: The Early Language Milestone Scale*. Tulsa: Modern Education Corporation.

Fluharty, N. B. (1974). *Fluharty Preschool Speech and Language Screening Test*. Teaching Resources Corp.

Haber, J. S., & Norris, M. L. (1983). The Texas Preschool Screening Inventory: A simple screening device for language and learning disorders. *Children's Health Care, 12* (1), 11–18.

Kulig, S. G., & Bakler, K. (1973). *Physician's Developmental Quick Screen for Speech Disorders*. Galveston, TX: University of Texas Medical Branch.

Striffler, N., & Willis, S. (1981). *Communication Screen*. Tucson, AZ: Communication Skills Builder.

Sturner, R. A., Layton, T. L., Evans, A. W., Funk, S. G., & Machon, M. W. (1994). Preschool speech and language screening: A review of currently available tests. *American Journal of Speech-Language Pathology, 3* (1), 25–36.

III. Audiologic Screening Guidelines—Adult Section

A. Rationale

This section contains sets of audiologic screening guidelines that pertain to any noninstitutionalized adult, 18 years old or older. (An ASHA ad hoc committee is preparing a separate document that addresses hearing screening in long-term care facilities.) Individuals who have been identified previously as having a hearing condition (disorder, impairment, or disability), or who are unable to participate in a conventional screening protocol are referred and recommended for immediate audiologic evaluation as deemed appropriate. Individuals participating in occupational hearing conservation programs are excluded.

Adult hearing screening programs are considered voluntary in nature. Competent adults by virtue of their presence at the screening site grant consent to receive the screening. Care needs to be exercised to ensure patient confidentiality and safety.

In the development of audiologic screening guidelines for adults, the Panel considered many adult-related issues including patient compliance, specific goals of adult screening, and the domains of screening for each hearing condition (disorder, impairment, and disability). Much of the discussion centered on models and issues is given in the "Report: Considerations in Screening Adults/Older Persons for Handicapping Hearing Impairment" (ASHA, 1992).

Hearing impairment is defined as unilateral or bilateral sensorineural and/or conductive hearing levels greater than 20 dB HL. Hearing impairment (i.e., loss or abnormality of psychological or physiological function) and/or hearing disability (i.e., restriction or lack of ability to perform an activity, resulting from an impairment) are prevalent chronic conditions among adults of all ages. It is recognized that hearing impairment increases as a function of age, especially for frequencies 2000 Hz and above. However, adults tend to ignore its effects, delay their decision to seek audiologic services, and demonstrate poor compliance with recommended treatments (Jupiter, 1989; Koike & Johnston, 1989; Schow, 1991; Trumble & Piterman, 1992; Weinstein & Ventry, 1983). Screening for hearing impairment and screening for hearing disability use different measures and, therefore, are presented separately in this document. Some persons with hearing impairment may not perceive any hearing disability. Conversely, some persons with minimal or no hearing impairment perceive considerable hearing disability. (Newman, Jacobson, Hug, & Sandridge, in press). For these reasons, screening for impairment and screening for disability are integral and equal parts of the total screening process.

Techniques for hearing screening of adults include case history, visual inspection, pure-tone screening, and screening by self-assessment of hearing disability. Pure-tone screening may be used to screen individuals for hearing impairment but cannot be used to screen for hearing disability. Self-report measures of perceived disability may be used to screen for hearing disability but may not be sensitive to hearing disorder or impairment. By developing separate guidelines for each hearing condition (disorder, impairment, and disability), the panel has addressed the conflict produced by screening for hearing impairment and disability with a single measure. Hearing screening guidelines that identify instruments and procedures for screening for hearing disorders, hearing impairment, and hearing disability permit development of appropriate recommendations for adults who demonstrate high levels of impairment with low levels of disability or low levels of impairment with high levels of disability (Schow, 1991). The Panel recommends screening for disorder, impairment, and disability. All recommendations and comments regarding the disposition of the adult patient screened for disorder, impairment, and disability are summarized on the Adult Hearing Screening Form (Appendix A).

1. Screening for Hearing Disorders—Adults

The purpose of screening for hearing disorder is to identify persons with significant otologic history or obvious anatomic abnormalities of the ear. Unless such conditions are currently under medical management, medical referral will be made.

The outline presented below contains the Panel's recommended guidelines for the development, supervision, and delivery of screening programs for ear disorders in adults. The Panel provides a discussion of important issues related to the rationale and assumptions underlying the recommendations. The Panel intends that this discussion section be considered fully prior to the implementation of the recommendations.

I. Personnel

Screening practitioners should be limited to:

A. Audiologists holding a Certificate of Clinical Competence (CCC-A) from the American Speech-Language-Hearing Association (ASHA) and state licensure where applicable (ASHA, 1996a).

B. Other medical practitioners.

II. Expected Outcomes

A. Identification of those persons who most likely have ear or other related conditions that require medical evaluation (ASHA, 1992).

B. Determination of candidacy for pure-tone air-conduction screening.

III. Clinical Indications

Screen individuals aged 18 years and older for hearing disorder as part of their voluntary participation in a screening protocol for hearing impairment or disability.

IV. Clinical Process

A. Conduct screening in a manner consistent with infection control and universal precautions (Ballachanda, Roeser, & Kemp, 1996; Jacobson, 1994; Kemp, Roeser, Pearson, & Ballachanda, 1995).

B. Obtain a case history in a face-to-face or paper and pencil format regarding: history of hearing loss, unilateral hearing loss, sudden or rapid progression of hearing loss, unilateral tinnitus, acute or chronic dizziness, recent drainage from the ear(s), and/or pain or discomfort in the ear(s) (U.S. Department of Health, Education and Welfare, Food and Drug Administration, 1977).

C. Visually inspect the outer ear to identify conditions warranting medical referral.

D. As training and scope of practice permits (ASHA, 1996b), conduct an otoscopic or video-otoscopic inspection to identify those individuals who may require medical referral (ASHA, 1992; Ballachanda, 1995). In addition, this inspection determines candidacy for pure-tone screening.

E. All hearing screening programs should include an educational component designed to provide individuals screened with information, in lay language, on the process of hearing screening, the likelihood of having a hearing disorder, and follow-up procedures.

V. Inappropriate Procedures

Immittance measures in lieu of direct visualization of the ear are not recommended because the incidence of middle ear disease is low in the adult population, and the diagnostic yield is negligible.

VI. Pass/Refer Criteria

A. Pass, if no positive results in either ear.

B. Refer, if any positive response for which the individual has not received medical attention is given in the case history.

C. Refer, if visual identification of any physical abnormality of the outer ear, or otoscopic identification of ear canal abnormality, or cerumen impaction.

VII. Follow-Up Procedures

Recommend immediate medical evaluation or cerumen management.

VIII. Setting/Instrument Specifications

A. Use an environment conducive to lighted otoscopy and interview confidentiality.

B. Use lighted otoscope or video-otoscope.

C. See recommended case history/visual/ otoscopic inspection forms (Appendix A).

IX. Documentation

Document identifying information, a case history, description of visual/otoscopic findings, and recommendations (Appendix A).

2. Screening for Hearing Impairment—Adults

A protocol for screening for hearing impairment is herein recommended. The recommended inclusion of the two other components of the adult screening program (screening for disorder and screening for disability) is considered essential given the known reticence of adults to acknowledge hearing impairment and/or hearing disability. Further, their low compliance in following recommendations for hearing assistance has been documented (Weinstein & Ventry, 1983). Results from the three components of the screening protocol together provide more useful information than single components for the purposes of counseling and referral.

The outline presented below contains recommended guidelines for the development, supervision, and delivery of screening programs for hearing impairment in adults. The Panel provides a discussion of important issues related to the rationale and assumptions underlying the recommendations. The Panel intends that this discussion section be considered fully prior to the implementation of the recommendations.

I. Personnel

Screening practitioners should be limited to:

A. Audiologists with a Certificate of Clinical Competence (CCC-A) from the American Speech-Language-Hearing Association (ASHA) and state licensure where applicable (ASHA, 1996a).

B. Speech-language pathologists with a Certificate of Clinical Competence (CCC-SLP) from the American Speech-Language-Hearing Association (ASHA) and state licensure where applicable (ASHA, 1996b).

C. Support personnel under the supervision of a certified audiologist (ASHA, 1981).

II. Expected Outcomes

Identification of those persons most likely to have hearing impairment that requires referral.

III. Clinical Indications

A. Screen as needed, requested, or when they have conditions that place them at risk for hearing impairment, such as recreational noise exposure, family history and concern of family member.

B. Screen at least every decade through age 50 and at 3-year intervals thereafter.

IV. Clinical Process

A. Instruct patients to respond in a specified manner (e.g., conventional audiometric techniques) each time auditory stimuli are perceived.

B. Position conventional earphones (or insert earphones) and present pure tones at 25 dB HL at the frequencies of 1000, 2000, and 4000 Hz. (See discussion.)

C. Record results on a form that contains demographic information and ear-specific and frequency-specific responses (Appendix A).

V. Pass/Refer Criteria

A. Pass if responses to pure-tone air-conduction stimuli at 25 dB HL at 1000, 2000, and 4000 Hz are obtained in both ears.

B. Refer if no response is observed at any frequency in either ear.

VI. Inappropriate Procedures

Methods using uncalibrated acoustic signals (e.g., whisper test, telephone hearing screening) or automated tests that are not conducted under the supervision of a certified audiologist.

VII. Follow-Up Procedures

A. Referral for hearing impairment involves brief counseling regarding hearing impairment. Counseling may result in a recommendation for audiologic evaluation, or discharge if an individual passed a hearing disability screen and declines audiologic evaluation.

B. If referrals from hearing impairment screen and from hearing disability screen are both indicated, recommend for audiologic evaluation.

VIII. Setting/Equipment Specifications

A. Conduct hearing screening in a clinical or natural environment conducive to obtaining reliable screening results.

B. Note that in screening environments, ambient noise levels may exceed ANSI (1991) standards for pure-tone threshold testing, but must be sufficiently low to allow accurate screening (See Table 1).

C. Meet ANSI S3.6-1996 requirements for either limited-range or narrow-range audiometers for all electroacoustic equipment.

D. Calibrate to ANSI specifications (ANSI S3.6-1996) regularly, at least once every year, following initial determination that the device meets all ANSI specifications. All the ANSI specifications, not just the sound pressure level, should be met.

E. Perform a daily listening check to rule out distortion, crosstalk, and intermittency, and to determine that no defects exist in major components.

F. Note that electroacoustic equipment should meet regulatory agency specification for electrical safety.

IX. Documentation

Use a form that contains identifying information, screening results, and recommendations, including the need for counseling or referral (Appendix A).

Discussion

Clinical Process

A uniform screening level of 25 dB HL at pure-tone frequencies of 1000, 2000, and 4000 Hz was selected. Hearing impairment in excess of 25 dB HL affects communication independent of age and reflects clinically significant hearing impairment. Goldstein's 1984 review of hearing loss surveys indicated that 28% of adults sampled had hearing losses exceeding 25 dB HL averaged across the frequencies of 1000, 2000, and 4000 Hz in the poorer ear.

It is recognized that the failure rate for hearing impairment increases as a function of age, especially for frequencies of 2000 Hz and higher (Gates, Cooper,

Table 1. ANSI S3.1-1991 maximum permissible ambient noise levels (MPANLs) for threshold testing to 0 dB HL at 1000, 2000, 4000 Hz and derivation of permissible noise levels for hearing screening at 25 dB HL.

Condition	Frequency in Hz		
	1000	2000	4000
1. MPANL ears not covered	14.0	8.5	9.0
2. Attenuation-supra-aural earphone	12.5	19.5	12.5
3. MPANL ears covered (Line 1 + Line 2)	26.5	28.0	34.5
4. Screening level	25	25	25
5. MPANL for screening (Line 3 + Line 4)	51.5	53.0	59.5
6. Attenuation-insert earphone[a]	33.5	33.0	40.5
7. MPANL ears plugged (Line 1 + Line 6)	47.5	41.5	49.5
8. Screening level	25	25	25
9. MPANL ears plugged (Line 7 + Line 8)	72.5	66.5	74.5

MPANLs in dB SPL for 1/3 octave bands. Add 5 dB for octave bands.
[a]From Frank & Williams (1993), rounded to nearest 0.5 dB.

Kannal, & Miller, 1990; Moscicki, Elkins, Baum, & McNamara, 1985). The panel recognizes that the referral rate will be higher for older adults with the uniform screening level of 25 dB HL. Schow (1991) reported that 27% of adults 18–59 years of age failed hearing screening at 25 dB HL using 1000, 2000, and 4000 Hz stimuli. Bess, Lichenstein, Logan, Burger, & Nelson (1989) found that 62% of their adult sample over age 65 had hearing losses greater than 25 dB HL averaged across the frequencies of 1000, 2000, and 4000 Hz. For those over age 60, Schow (1991) found that 77% of them failed to hear at least one of the stimuli at 25 dB HL. Additionally, Schow (1995) has reported that mean scores on the Self-Assessment of Communication (SAC) move out of the normal range as pure-tone sensitivity exceeds 25–30 dB at 1000 Hz and 2000 Hz. Thus, though a higher referral rate for older adults is anticipated, the uniform screening level of 25 dB HL was adopted because hearing impairments exceeding 25 dB HL can affect communication regardless of age.

Even mild hearing losses have significant impact on health and well-being. Bess, Lichtenstein, & Logan (1991) reported that each 10 dB decrease in hearing sensitivity resulted in a statistically significant change on the overall Sickness Impact Profile (SIP) (Gilson et al., 1975). For these reasons, the Panel recommends that screening for hearing impairment should be included as part of health screening programs that occur in the community or as a part of routine physical examinations.

Hearing screening with pure-tone stimuli has shown good sensitivity and specificity in identifying hearing losses exceeding a predetermined screening level (e.g., 25 dB HL) and, conversely, in ruling out hearing losses for individuals having thresholds better than the selected screening criterion. Using an Audioscope™, Bienvenue, Michael, Chaffinish, and Ziegler (1985) obtained sensitivity values of 93% to 98% and specificities of 70% to 88% when compared to threshold tests performed with a conventional audiometer. The higher sensitivity and specificity occurred when the audiometric tests were compared to the second screen for those who failed the first screening test. Frank and Petersen (1987) used the Audioscope™ and a conventional audiometer for screening and then compared screening results to conventional audiometric test findings across the frequency range of 500 through 4000 Hz. They found overall sensitivity to be 90% and 92%, and specificity to be 93% and 94% for the Audioscope™ and conventional audiometer, respectively. Alvord (1993) compared results using an Otoscreen™ in physicians' offices against threshold results obtained in a conventional test booth. He found screening sensitivity ranging from 95% to 99% and specificity from 78% to 99% across the frequency region of 500 through 4000 Hz. Specificity was lowest at 500 Hz, attributed to the noise levels at 500 Hz in the physicians' offices.

3. Screening for Hearing Disability—Adults

Screening for hearing disability requires self-assessment measures having strong internal consistency/reliability and test-retest reliability. A protocol for screening for hearing disability is herein recommended. The recommended inclusion of the two other components of the adult screening program (screening for disorder and impairment) is considered essential given the known reticence of adults to acknowledge hearing impairment and/or hearing disability. Further, their low compliance in following recommendations for hearing assistance has been documented. Results from the three components of the screening protocol together provide more useful information than single components for the purposes of counseling and referral.

The outline presented below contains the Panel's recommended guidelines for the development, supervision, and delivery of screening programs for hearing disability in adults. The Panel provides a discussion of important issues related to the rationale and assumptions underlying the recommendations. The Panel intends that this discussion section be considered fully prior to the implementation of the recommendations.

I. Personnel

Limit screening practitioners to:

A. Audiologists with a Certificate of Clinical Competence (CCC-A) from the American Speech-Language-Hearing Association (ASHA) and state licensure where applicable (ASHA, 1996a).

B. Speech-language pathologists with a Certificate of Clinical Competence (CCC-SLP) from the American Speech-Language-Hearing Association (ASHA) and state licensure where applicable (ASHA, 1996b).

C. Support personnel under the supervision of a certified audiologist (ASHA, 1981).

II. Expected Outcomes

Identification of those persons most likely to have hearing disabilities that interfere with their social, educational, vocational performance, and communication.

III. Clinical Indications

A. Screen adults as needed, requested, or when they have conditions that place them at risk for hearing disability (e.g., family history, concern of family member).

B. Screen at least every decade through age 50 and at 3-year intervals thereafter.

IV. Clinical Process

A. Use hearing disability measures that are reliable and valid.

B. Examples of commonly used hearing disability screening instruments include: the Hearing Handicap Inventory for the Elderly – Screening version (HHIE-S; Ventry & Weinstein, 1983), and the Self-Assessment of Communication (SAC; Schow & Nerbonne, 1982).

C. Administer these measures in a face-to-face interview format; however, if the instruments have been shown to be psychometrically robust using written responses, these indices may be administered using a paper-pencil format.

D. Record the responses on a form that contains demographic information and the score on the hearing disability screening measure (Appendix A).

V. Inappropriate Procedures

Do not use measures that do not offer published data regarding internal consistency/reliability, test-retest reliability, and pass/refer criteria.

Table 1. HHIE-S Raw Score Handicap Range and Posthoc Probability of Hearing Impairment (Lichtenstein, Bess, & Logan, 1988)

Raw Score*		Posthoc Probability
0–8	No Handicap/No Referral	13%
10–24	Mild- to-Moderate Handicap	50%
26–40	Severe Handicap	84%

* Refer if score equals 10 or greater.

VI. Pass/Refer Criteria

Pass/refer criteria are indicated in Tables 1 and 2.

VII. Follow-Up Procedures

A. Recommendations may involve counseling, audiologic assessment, and/or other examinations or services.

B. Counseling includes informing the person that his or her score on the hearing disability questionnaire falls outside the established norms and may result in recommendation for audiologic evaluation, or discharge if the adult passed hearing impairment screen and declines audiologic evaluation.

C. If referred based on both the hearing disability and hearing impairment screening results, recommend for audiologic evaluation.

VIII. Setting/Instrument Specifications

A. Use any quiet environment conducive to interview and confidentiality.

B. See hearing disability screening questionnaire (Appendix B).

IX. Documentation

Complete hearing disability screening questionnaire (Appendix B).

Discussion

Clinical Process

The Self Assessment of Communication (SAC) (Schow & Nerbonne, 1982) and the Hearing Handicap Inventory for the Elderly–Screening Version (HHIE-S) (Ventry & Weinstein, 1983) are self-assessment measures of hearing disability that appear to be psychometrically robust. For example, the HHIE-S shows a test-retest reliability of 0.84 (Ventry & Weinstein, 1983). The SAC shows a test-retest reliability of 0.80 (Schow & Nerbonne, 1982).

The issue of assessing the criterion validity (comparing the results of a screening measure to some independent and valid measure) is complex. Specifically, one must choose an appropriate criterion measure. To assess criterion validity, it has been suggested that global measures of the impact of a disorder be employed; for example, SIP (Gilson et al., 1975).

The SIP consists of 136 items that are grouped into 12 subscales that assess the effects of sickness on the physical, psychosocial, and other spheres of function. Bess, Lichtenstein, Logan, & Burger (1989) and Bess, Lichtenstein, & Logan (1991) compared scores on the HHIE-S to scores on the SIP. The authors reported that: (a) the mean SIP score for those elderly subjects with even mild hearing impairment exceeded the SIP scores of heart-transplant patients; and (b) subjects with severe hearing handicaps (HHIE-S

Table 2. SAC, SAC Scoring and Interpretation (Schow, Smedley, & Longhurst, 1990)

Raw Score*	Handicap
10–18	Normal—No handicap
19–26	Slight handicap
27–38	Mild-moderate handicap
39–50	Severe handicap

* Refer if score equals 19 or greater.

Table 3. Mean Sickness Impact Profile (SIP) scores stratified by results from the Hearing Handicap Inventory for the Elderly (Bess, Lichtenstein, Logan, & Burger, 1989, p. 801).

HHIE-S score	0 – 8	10 – 24	26 – 40
	n = 95	*n* = 45	*n* = 13
SIP Scale	*Mean* (<u>SD</u>)	*Mean* (<u>SD</u>)	*Mean* (<u>SD</u>)
Physical Dimension	4.1 (8.3)	8.1 (9.6)	18.5 (12.5)
Psychosocial Dimension	4.0 (6.2)	10.3 (12.6)	22.2 (18.3)
Overall	5.8 (7.8)	10.8 (10.4)	23.0 (14.7)

score exceeding 24 points) demonstrated greater effects of hearing impairment in the physical and psychosocial content domains than those subjects classified as having no handicap on the HHIE-S (Table 3). Additionally, the authors reported that each 10 dB increase in hearing loss was associated with a 2.8 point increase in the SIP physical dimension score. The same 10 dB increase was associated with 2.0 and 1.3 point increases in the psychosocial and overall scores of the HHIE-S, respectively.

Others have compared the results of hearing disability screening tools with degraded word recognition tasks (Fire, Lesner, & Newman, 1991; Gatehouse, 1991; Jerger, Oliver, & Pirozzolo, 1990; Matthews, Lee, Mills, & Schum, 1990). The extent that estimates of speech recognition in background noise or distorted speech materials (e.g., accelerated speech; Gatehouse, 1990a, 1990b) can be used as a criterion measure compared to measures of hearing disability is not clear. For example, Jerger et al. (1990) administered the Synthetic Sentence Identification (SSI) test, the Speech Perception in Noise (SPIN) test, the Dichotic Sentence Identification (DSI) test, and the HHIE of Ventry & Weinstein (1982) to a group of elderly subjects. The authors reported significantly poorer HHIE scores for those subjects classified as having central auditory pathway disorders as determined by the speech test results. Similar findings have been reported by Fire et al. (1991). Matthews and associates (1990) observed correlations of 0.63 and 0.47 on the SPIN test (+8 signal-to-noise ratio) and total scores on the HHIE for the right ear and left ear, respectively.

The validity of the SAC was evaluated by establishing the level of association between the SAC and the Rating Scale for Each Ear (RSEE). The RSEE is a self-report measure developed at Gallaudet College (Schein, Gentile, & Haase, 1970) wherein subjects report, for each ear, whether their hearing is good, whether they have a little or considerable trouble hearing, or whether they are deaf. The Pearson correlation coefficient was 0.66 between the RSEE and the SAC. Additionally, the relationships between audiometric (impairment) measures such as pure-tone average (PTA) and speech-recognition threshold (SRT) and the SAC have been evaluated. The correlations were 0.78 and 0.80 for PTA and SRT respectively (Schow, 1995).

A general observation is that the performance characteristics of the SAC and HHIE-S for the identification of hearing impairment are equivalent for individuals 65 years and older (Schow, 1995). Additionally, the correlation coefficient between scores on the SAC and the HHIE-S has been reported to be high, 0.918 (Frank, Shostek, & Blood, 1989).

B. References

Alvord, L. S. (1993). Miniature audiometric devices: Are they clinically accurate? *Hearing Instruments, 44* (6), 24–25.

American National Standards Institute. (1996). *Specification for audiometers* (ANSI S3.6-1996). New York: ANSI.

American National Standards Institute. (1991). *Maximum permissible ambient noise levels for audiometric test rooms.* (ANSI S3.1-1991). New York: ANSI.

American Speech-Language-Hearing Association. (1981, March). Guidelines for the employment and utilization of supportive personnel. *Asha, 23,* 165–169.

American Speech-Language-Hearing Association. (1992, August). Report: Considerations in screening adults/older persons for handicapping hearing impairment. *Asha, 34,* 81–87.

American Speech-Language-Hearing Association. (1996a, Spring). Scope of practice in audiology. *Asha, 38* (Suppl. 16), 12–15.

American Speech-Language-Hearing Association. (1996b, Spring). Scope of practice in speech-language pathology. *Asha, 38* (Suppl. 16), 1–4.

Ballachanda, B. B. (1995). *The human ear canal.* San Diego, CA: Singular Publishing Group.

Ballachanda, B. B., Roeser, R. J., & Kemp, R. J. (1996). Control and prevention of disease transmission in audiology practice. *American Journal of Audiology, 5* (1), 74–82.

Bess, F. H., Lichtenstein, M. J., & Logan, S. A. (1991). Making hearing impairment functionally relevant: Linkages between hearing disability and handicap. *Acta Otolaryngologica,* (Suppl. 476), 226–231.

Bess, F. H., Lichtenstein, M. J., Logan, S. A., & Burger, M. C. (1989). Comparing criteria of hearing impairment in the elderly: A functional approach. *Journal of Speech and Hearing Research, 32,* 795–802.

Bess, F. H., Lichtenstein, M. J., Logan, S. A., Burger, M. C., & Nelson, E. (1989). Hearing impairment as detriment of function in the elderly. *Journal of the American Geriatric Society, 37,* 921–928.

Bienvenue, G. R., Michael, P. L., Chaffinish, J. C., & Ziegler, J. (1985). The Audioscope™: A clinical tool for otoscopic and audiometric examination. *Ear and Hearing, 6,* 251–254.

Fire, K. M., Lesner, S. A., & Newman, C. (1991). Hearing handicap as a function of central auditory processing abilities in the elderly. *American Journal of Otology, 12,* 105–108.

Frank, T., & Petersen, D. R. (1987). Accuracy of a 40 dB HL Audioscope™ and audiometer screening for adults. *Ear and Hearing, 8,* 180–183.

Frank, T., Shostek, C., & Blood, I. (1989). *HHIE-S and SAC screening for hearing impairment.* Convention of the American Speech-Language-Hearing Association, St. Louis.

Frank, T., & Williams, D. L. (1993). Effects of background noise on earphone thresholds. *Journal of the American Academy of Audiology, 4,* 201–212.

Gatehouse, S. (1990a). The contribution of central auditory factors to auditory disability. *Acta Otolaryngologica,* (Suppl. 476), 182–188.

Gatehouse, S. (1990b). The role of nonauditory factors in measured and self-reported disability. *Acta Otolaryngologica,* (Suppl. 476), 249–256.

Gates, G. A., Cooper, J. C., Kannal, W. B., & Miller, N. J. (1990). Hearing in the elderly: The Framingham Cohort, 1983–1985. *Ear and Hearing, 11,* 247–256.

Gilson, B. S., Gilson, J. S., Bergner, M., Bobbitt, R. A., Kressel, S., Pollard, W. E., & Vesselago, M. (1975). The Sickness Impact Profile: Development of an outcome measure of health care. *American Journal of Public Health, 65,* 1304–1310.

Goldstein, D. P. (1984, September). Hearing impairment, hearing aids and audiology. *Asha, 26,* 5–31.

Jacobson, G. (1994). Infection control. In *Development and management of audiology practices* (pp. 89–90). Rockville, MD: ASHA.

Jerger, J., Oliver, T., Pirozzolo, F. (1990). Impact of central auditory processing disorder and cognitive deficit on the self-assessment of hearing handicap in the elderly. *Journal of the American Academy of Audiology, 1,* 75–81.

Jupiter, T. (1989). A community hearing screening program for the elderly. *Hearing Journal, 42,* 14–17.

Kemp, R. J., Roeser, R. J., Pearson, D. W., & Ballachanda, B. B. (1995). *Infection control for the profession of audiology and speech-language pathology.* Chesterfield, MO: Oaktree Products.

Koike, K. J., & Johnston, A. P. (1989). Follow-up survey of the elderly who failed a hearing screening protocol. *Ear and Hearing, 10,* 250–253.

Lichtenstein, M. J., Bess, F. H., & Logan, S. A. (1988). Diagnostic performance of the Hearing Handicap Inventory for the Elderly (Screening version) against differing definitions of hearing loss. *Ear and Hearing, 9,* 209–211.

Matthews, L. J., Lee, F. S., Mills, J. H., & Schum, D. J. (1990). Audiometric and subjective assessment of hearing handicap. *Archives of Otolaryngology—Head and Neck Surgery, 116,* 1325–1330.

Moscicki, E. K., Elkins, E. F., Baum, H. M., & McNamara, P. M. (1985). Hearing loss in the elderly: An epidemiologic study of the Framingham heart study cohort. *Ear and Hearing, 6,* 184–190.

Newman, C. W., Jacobson, G. P., Hug, G. A., & Sandridge, S. A. (In press). Perceived hearing handicaps by patients with unilateral or mixed hearing loss. *Annals of Otology, Rhinology and Laryngology.*

Schein, J., Gentile, A., & Haase, K. (1970). Development and evaluation of an expanded hearing loss scale questionnaire. *Vital and Health Statistics, 2,* 37.

Schow, R. L. (1991). Considerations in selecting and validating an adult/elderly hearing screening protocol. *Ear and Hearing, 12,* 337–348.

Schow, R. L. (1995). *Status and future of SAC and SOAC: Psychometric studies.* Presented at the International Collegium of Rehabilitative Audiology, Goteborg, Sweden, May 1995.

Schow, R. L., & Nerbonne, M. A. (1982). Communication Screening Profile: Use with elderly clients. *Ear and Hearing, 3,* 134–147.

Schow, R. L., Smedley, T. C., & Longhurst, T. M. (1990). Self-assessment and impairment in adult/elderly hearing screening—Recent data and new perspectives. *Ear and Hearing, 11,* 17S–27S.

Trumble, S. C., & Piterman, L. (1992). Hearing loss in the elderly. *Medical Journal of Australia, 157,* 400–404.

U.S. Department of Health, Education, and Welfare, Food and Drug Administration. (1977, February 15). Hearing aid devices: Professional and patient labeling and conditions for sale (48 *Federal Register,* Title 21. Chapter 1, Sub-Chapter H, Part 801, pp. 9286–9296).

Ventry, I., & Weinstein, B. (1982). The Hearing Handicap Inventory for the Elderly: A new tool. *Ear and Hearing, 3,* 128–134.

Ventry, I., & Weinstein, B. (1983). Identification of elderly people with hearing problems. *Asha, 25,* 37–42.

Weinstein, B., & Ventry, I. (1983). Audiometric correlates of the Hearing Handicap Inventory for the Elderly. *Journal of Speech and Hearing Disorders, 48,* 379–384.

Appendix A. Hearing Screening (Adults)

Name _____ Date _____

Birth Date _____ Age _____ Gender: M   F

Screening Unit/Examiner _____ Calibration Date _____

Case History—circle appropriate answers

Do you think you have a hearing loss?	Yes	No
Have hearing aid(s) ever been recommended for you?	Yes	No
Is your hearing better in one ear?	Yes	No

If yes, which is the better ear?   Right   Left

Have you ever had a sudden or rapid progression of hearing loss?	Yes	No

If yes, which ear?   Right   Left

Do you have ringing or noises in your ears?	Yes	No

If yes,   Right   Left   Both

Do you consider dizziness to be a problem for you?	Yes	No
Have you had recent drainage from your ear(s)?	Yes	No

If yes,   Right   Left

Do you have pain or discomfort in your ear(s)?	Yes	No

If yes,   Right   Left

Have you received medical consultation for any of the above conditions?	Yes	No

PASS   **REFER**

Visual/Otoscopic Inspection

PASS   **REFER**   **Right**   **Left**

Referral for cerumen management _____ Referral for medical evaluation _____

Pure-Tone Screen (25 dB HL)   (R = Response, NR = No Response)

Frequency	1000	2000	4000 Hz
Right Ear			
Left Ear			

PASS   **REFER**

Hearing-Disability Index

Score: HHIE-S_____ SAC _____ Other _____ Score _____

PASS   **REFER**

Discharge   ___ Medical Examination   ___Counsel

               ___ Cerumen Management   ___Audiologic Evaluation

Comments _____

_____

Patient Signature _____ Date _____

Appendix B. Self-Assessment of Communication
(SAC; Schow & Nerbonne, 1982)

Please respond by circling the appropriate number ranging from 1 to 5, for the following questions. If you have a hearing aid, please fill out the form according to how you communicate when aid is *not* in use.

1 = almost never (or never); 2 = occasionally (about one-quarter of the time); 3 = about half of the time; 4 = frequently (about three-quarters of the time); 5 = practically always (or always).

Various Communication Situations

1. Do you experience communication difficulties in situations when speaking with one other person? (For example: at home, at work, in a social situation, with a waitress, a store clerk, a boss, etc.)

    1   2   3   4   5

2. Do you experience communication difficulties in situations when conversing with a small group of several persons? (For example: with friends or family, co-workers, in meetings or casual conversations, over dinner, or while playing cards, etc.).

    1   2   3   4   5

3. Do you experience communication difficulties while listening to someone speak to a large group? (For example, at church or in a civic meeting, in a fraternal or women's club, at an educational lecture, etc.)

    1   2   3   4   5

4. Do you experience communication difficulties while participating in various types of entertainment? (For example: TV, radio, plays, night clubs, musical entertainment, etc.)

    1   2   3   4   5

5. Do you experience communication difficulties when you are in an unfavorable listening environment? (For example: at a noisy party, where there is background music, when riding in an auto or a bus, when someone whispers or talks from across the room, etc.)

    1   2   3   4   5

6. Do you experience communication difficulties when using or listening to various communication devices? (For example: telephone, telephone ring, doorbell, public address system, warning signals, alarms, etc.)

    1   2   3   4   5

Feelings About Communication

7. Do you feel that any difficulty with your hearing limits or hampers your personal or social life?

    1   2   3   4   5

8. Does any problem or difficulty with your hearing upset you?

    1   2   3   4   5

Other People

9. Do others suggest that you have a hearing problem?

    1   2   3   4   5

10. Do others leave you out of conversations or become annoyed because of your hearing?

    1   2   3   4   5

Raw Score _____ (total of circled numbers; normal range: 10–18)

Score Interpretation (Schow, Smedley, & Longhurst, 1990):

Raw score	Handicap range
10–18	Normal-no handicap
19–26	Slight handicap
27–38	Mild-moderate handicap
39–50	Severe handicap

Appendix C. Hearing Handicap Inventory for the Elderly
Screening Version (HHIE-S; Ventry & Weinstein, 1983)

Please check "yes," "no," or "sometimes" in response to each of the following items. Do not skip a question if you avoid a situation because of a hearing problem. If you use a hearing aid, please answer the way you hear without the aid.

E = emotional   S = social   "No" response = 0   "Sometimes" = 2   "Yes" = 4

			Yes	Sometimes	No
E	1.	Does a hearing problem cause you to feel embarrassed when you meet new people?			
E	2.	Does a hearing problem cause you to feel frustrated when talking to members of your family?			
S	3.	Do you have difficulty hearing when someone speaks in a whisper?			
E	4.	Do you feel handicapped by a hearing problem?			
S	5.	Does a hearing problem cause you difficulty when visiting friends, relatives, or neighbors?			
S	6.	Does a hearing problem cause you to attend religious services less often than you would like?			
E	7.	Does a hearing problem cause you to have arguments with family members?			
S	8.	Does a hearing problem cause you difficulty when listening to TV or radio?			
E	9.	Do you feel that any difficulty with your hearing limits or hampers your personal or social life?			
S	10.	Does a hearing problem cause you difficulty when in a restaurant with relatives or friends?			
	Score ——————				

HHIE-S Score Interpretation (Lichtenstein, Bess, & Logan, 1988)

Raw Score	Handicap Range	Posthoc Prob. of Hearing Impairment
0–8	No handicap	13%
10–24	Mild-moderate handicap	50%
26–40	Severe handicap	84%

Appendix D. Bibliography

American Speech-Language-Hearing Association. (1992, March). External auditory canal examination and cerumen management. *Asha, 34-*(Suppl. 7), 22–24.

American Speech-Language-Hearing Association. (1993, March). Definitions of communication disorders and variations. *Asha, 35* (Suppl. 10), 24–32.

American Speech-Language-Hearing Association. (1996, March). Clinical practice by certificate holders in the profession in which they are not certified. *Asha, 38* (Suppl. 16), 11–12.

Davis, J. M., Elfenbein, J., Schum, R., & Bentler, R. A. (1986). Effects of mild and moderate hearing impairments on language, education and psychosocial behavior of children. *Journal of Speech and Hearing Disorders, 51*, 53–62.

Greenberg, M. T. (1983). Family stress and child competence: The effects of early intervention for families with deaf infants. *American Annals of the Deaf, 128*, 407–417.

Greenberg, M. T. (1984). Early invention: Outcomes and issues. *Topics in Early Childhood and Special Education, 3*, 1–19.

Greenberg, M. T., Calderon, R., & Kusche, C. (1984). Early intervention using simultaneous communication with deaf infants: The effect on communication development. *Child Development, 55*, 607–616.

Harford, E. R., Bess, F. H., Bluestone, C. D., & Klein, J. O., (Eds.). (1978). *Impedance screening for middle ear disease in children.* New York: Grune & Stratton.

Kuhl, P. K., Williams, K. A., Lacerda, F., Stephens, K. N., & Lindbloom, B. (1992). Linguistic experience alters phonetics perception in infants by six months of age. *Science, 255*, 606–608.

Levitt, H., McGarr, N. S., & Geffner, D. (1987). Development of language and communication skills in hearing-impaired children. *ASHA Monographs, 26*.

Margolis, R. H., & Heller, J. W. (1987). Screening tympanometry: Criteria for medical referral. *Audiology, 26*, 197–208.

Moeller, M., Osberger, M., & Eccarius, M. (1986). Receptive language skills. In M. Osberger (Ed.), Language and learning skills in hearing-impaired students. *ASHA Monographs, 23*, 41–53.

Nozza, R. J. (1996). Pediatric hearing screening. In F. N. Martin & J. G. Clark (Eds.), *Hearing care for children* (pp. 95–114). Needham Heights, MA: Allyn & Bacon.

Roush, J. (1992). Screening school-age children. In F. H. Bess & J. W. Hall III (Eds.), *Screening children for auditory function* (pp. 297–313). Nashville: Bill Wilkerson Center Press.

Stein, L. (1995). The volunteer audiologist. *Audiology Today, 7*, 17–18.

Turner, R. G. (1990, September). Recommended guidelines for infant hearing screening: Analysis. *Asha*, 57–61, 66.

U.S. Public Health Service. (1994). *The clinician's handbook of preventive services* (pp. 176–179). Alexandria, VA: International Medical Publishing.

Yoshinaga-Itano, C. (1995). Efficacy of early identification and early intervention. *Seminars in Hearing, 16*, 115–123.